Air Fryer Diet Recipes for Beginners

© Copyright 2023 by Darren Carr

Copyright © 2023 by Darren Carr
All rights reserved. No part of this book may be reproduced, scanned,
or distributed in any printed or electronic form without permission.

First Edition: November 2023

Cover: Illustration made by Mary C.

Printed in the United States of America

TABLE OF CONTENTS

Dedicated to all my friends and to all the people
who gave me their help.
Thanks a lot
Thanks to all of you for your confidence
in my qualities and what I do.
Darren Carr

CHAPTER 1

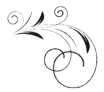

INTRODUCTION TO THE AIR FRYER DIET

Understanding the Concept of the Air Fryer Diet

The air fryer diet is transforming home cooking and introducing a healthier way to enjoy fried foods. At its core, this diet simply utilizes an air fryer to prepare wholesome, low-carb meals that support weight loss goals. By harnessing rapid air circulation technology, the air fryer allows you to eliminate excess oil and fat from recipes while still achieving crispy textures and rich flavors. Adopting this innovative appliance empowers you to take control of your diet and make positive changes.

When beginning the air fryer diet, it is helpful to understand the core principles behind this approach. First and foremost, the air fryer reduces oil and fat content substantially compared to traditional frying methods. The superheated air quickly cooks food from all sides, eliminating the need for submerging ingredients in oil. This significantly cuts calories and fat intake. While not completely oil-free, air frying uses teaspoons instead of cups of oil to prepare dishes.

In addition, the air fryer diet focuses on lean proteins, fresh produce, and complex carbohydrates. Meals feature poultry, fish, eggs, legumes, vegetables, fruits, whole grains, nuts and healthy fats like olive or avocado oil. Refined carbs, added sugars, salty snacks, and fatty cuts of red meat are consumed sparingly. Home cooked meals maximize nutrition while keeping portions and calories controlled.

Unlike restrictive fad diets, the air fryer diet provides flexibility and versatility. You can air fry everything from breakfast staples like omelets and avocado toast to main courses such as salmon, chicken wings, or eggplant parmesan. Side dishes like roasted vegetables, zucchini fries and Brussels sprouts also shine. The appliance allows you to enjoy crispy textures and rich flavors using little to no oil, keeping calories and fat intake under control. From Tex-Mex dishes to Mediterranean fare, the possibilities are endless.

Several factors make the air fryer diet more manageable and sustainable than extreme low-calorie diets. Firstly, the satisfying meals prevent hunger and cravings which often derail diets. Protein and fiber keep you fuller for longer while stabilizing blood sugar. Secondly, the varied recipes mean you don't tire of bland "diet food." Thirdly, the hands-off nature of the air fryer and easier cleanup helps you stick to home cooking. Above all, the ability to enjoy crispy, flavorful foods without excess oil or calories reduces feelings of deprivation.

When followed consistently, the air fryer diet provides numerous benefits beyond just weight loss. The abundance of lean proteins, fresh produce and healthy fats improves overall nutrition. Monitoring carbohydrate intake helps stabilize blood sugar and insulin, the key hormone regulating fat storage. Relying on home cooking instead of takeout reduces sodium, preservatives and additives. Most importantly, this diet helps reboot tastebuds and cravings to prefer natural whole foods over processed items.

The air fryer makes it easy to enjoy delicious plant-based dishes, a boon for vegetarians and vegans. It's perfect for crisping up tofu, preparing veggie burgers, roasting cauliflower or making vegan "wings." Meatless proteins like legumes, nuts, eggs and dairy provide satisfying protein options. The focus on produce highlights the many vegetables and fruits that shine through air frying. With a little creativity, the air fryer diet caters to diverse needs and preferences.

While the air fryer cannot work miracles on its own, it is an invaluable asset for healthy eating and weight management. This versatile appliance eliminates the biggest obstacles that derail many diets – lack of variety, low satiety and cravings. With an arsenal of air fryer recipes, you can whip up an array of meals beyond typical diet fare. From breakfast tacos to vegetable curries, kebabs to frittatas, the possibilities are endless. The satisfaction provided by delicious, home-cooked meals makes it easier to stick to your nutritional targets.

Several characteristics of the air fryer diet facilitate safe, sustainable weight loss. Firstly, the focus on protein and fresh produce provides nutrients vital for fat burning and muscle synthesis. Secondly, the reduced carb intake and low oil usage create a moderate daily calorie deficit to spur fat loss. Thirdly, the satisfying recipes and properly portioned meals prevent hunger, cravings and bingeing. By reducing body fat and revealing lean muscle, the air fryer diet provides more effective weight loss compared to extreme crash diets.

Embarking on the air fryer diet requires some advance preparation to set yourself up for success. Gradually reduce processed carbs, added sugars and fried takeout while increasing whole, nutritious foods. This eases the adjustment period when you fully cut back on high-carb fare. Next, invest in a quality air fryer suited for your cooking needs and kitchen space. Finally, cultivate a positive, motivated mindset focused on your health goals. Monitoring your eating habits, energy and cravings helps you understand the diet's impact. With the right preparation, the air fryer diet can transform your body and life.

In summary, the air fryer diet centers around preparing lean, low-carb meals in this innovative appliance to reduce fat and facilitate weight loss. With a focus on proteins, fresh produce and complex carbs, it provides nutrition without deprivation. While requiring some lifestyle adjustments, the versatile air fryer empowers you to enjoy fried favorites without guilt. Adopting this diet with proper diligence and commitment can truly transform your health, waistline and relationship with food.

The Benefits of Low-Carb and Budget-Friendly Meals

Transitioning to a low-carb diet can seem intimidating at first, but embracing more wholesome, budget-conscious eating provides tremendous benefits for your health, waistline, and wallet. This lifestyle empowers you to take control of your food choices so you can look and feel your absolute best.

One of the biggest perks of low-carb eating is steady, sustainable weight loss. When you cut back on sugar, refined grains, and starchy foods, you stabilize blood sugar and insulin levels. This kickstarts fat burning and curbs cravings that lead to overeating. Even a modest reduction in carbs coupled with mindful calorie control can lead to incredible results over time. Shedding just a few pounds can dramatically reduce your risk for obesity-related diseases like heart disease and diabetes.

Going low-carb doesn't mean depriving yourself of delicious food or feeling hungry all the time. In fact, healthy fats and proteins provide satiety between meals so you feel satisfied on fewer calories. And you still get to enjoy plenty of fiber-rich fruits and vegetables, like leafy greens, broccoli, berries, and more. Planning meals around these nourishing whole foods provides steady energy levels rather than spikes and crashes from refined carbs.

Cutting back on packaged, processed items also saves money at the grocery store. Sticking to basic whole ingredients that you prepare yourself keeps food budgets reasonable. Opting for cheaper cuts of meat and buying frozen or canned produce allows you to keep eating well without breaking the bank. With a little creativity in the kitchen, you can whip up inexpensive yet totally crave-worthy meals.

Your cooking skills will grow exponentially when you begin preparing more dishes at home. Following tempting low-carb recipes helps make healthy eating enjoyable rather than a chore. You may find joy in creating tasty meals for yourself and your family. Home cooking also allows you to control exactly what goes into your food. This empowerment will only further motivate your health journey.

Beyond physical benefits, transitioning to a low-carb lifestyle can greatly impact your mental health and outlook, especially if you are living with obesity or diabetes. Shedding excess weight and controlling blood sugar reduces joint pain, boosts mobility, and increases energy levels. You will likely find yourself feeling more motivated to move your body and participate in activities you love. Exercise becomes enjoyable rather than a tiring feat.

As your health improves, your confidence will skyrocket. You may notice a sunnier outlook overall without excess blood sugar wreaking havoc on your moods. Clearer skin, better sleep, and a boosted libido are other common perks of low-carb eating. Simply feeling comfortable in your own body again is invaluable.

Committing to more home cooking and fewer carbs provides health benefits for the whole family. Teaching kids about nutrition early on sets them up for success. Plus, low-carb swaps like cauliflower rice and zucchini noodles are stealthy ways to increase veggie intake. Shared family meals also offer a chance to disconnect from devices and connect with each other.

While behavior changes take time and patience, embracing a low-carb lifestyle puts you firmly on the path toward your health goals. With some planning and creativity, you can find budget-friendly ways to cook nourishing meals at home. This lifestyle empowers you to take control of your diet and reap amazing benefits for body and mind. Each small step brings you closer to becoming your healthiest, happiest self.

The Role of the Air Fryer in a Healthy Lifestyle

The air fryer has emerged as one of the most versatile and beneficial kitchen appliances for pursuing a healthy lifestyle. With its ability to crisp and "fry" foods with minimal oil, the air fryer allows you to reduce the fat and calories in traditionally unhealthy fried items. But the usefulness of the air fryer goes beyond faux-frying. This handy appliance can assist with meal planning, weight management, and nutrition in numerous ways.

Introducing the air fryer into your kitchen routine supports healthy eating habits. The air fryer's compact size and ease of use makes it convenient to cook fresh, wholesome meals at home. The rapid air technology heats up swiftly, cooking ingredients in a fraction of the time of a conventional oven. This allows you to prepare dishes quickly even on your busiest days. The small capacity of most air fryer baskets encourages properly portioned meals, unlike giant ovens that encourage oversized portions. When you're equipped with an arsenal of go-to air fryer recipes, resisting the temptation of takeout or processed convenience foods becomes much more manageable.

Another advantage of the air fryer is its ability to transform traditionally unhealthy fried foods into healthier versions. Southern fried chicken, crispy French fries, chicken parm—you name it, the air fryer can give it a guilt-free makeover. By using just a spritz of oil or none at all, you eliminate up to 80% of the fat and calories versus deep frying, while keeping the same delicious flavor and crunch. The air fryer allows you to enjoy your favorite comfort foods and still meet your health goals. Additionally, the air fryer excels at cooking frozen foods from their raw state with no oil required. You can conveniently prepare frozen foods like chicken nuggets, sweet potato fries or fish sticks from their healthier, additive-free frozen forms.

The versatility of the air fryer also promotes healthy eating through all of its cooking capabilities beyond air frying. Almost anything you'd normally prepare in your oven or on the stovetop can be made in your air fryer. The technology uses superheated, rapidly circulating air to mimic the results of frying, baking, grilling, roasting or broiling. From crisping up brussels sprouts or broccoli to roasting salmon fillets or whole chickens, the options are endless. The speedy cooking times help preserve nutrients that might otherwise be lost using traditional cooking methods.

Furthermore, the air fryer allows you to get creative with recipes that promote fruits, vegetables, lean proteins and healthy fats—all staples of a balanced diet. For instance, air fryer recipes enable you to whip up veggie-based "fries" from carrots, zucchini or eggplant for a colorful, nutrient-packed substitution to traditional fries. Meals like air fried tofu veggie bowls and cauliflower "wings" also fit into several dietary lifestyles like vegetarian, vegan, gluten-free and more. Even meat lovers can use the air fryer for recipes like turkey meatballs, bacon-wrapped pork tenderloin or lemon pepper salmon. It caters to all types of healthy eaters.

For individuals focused on weight loss, the air fryer can be an invaluable asset. As mentioned earlier, the oil-free cooking process significantly slashes calories compared to deep frying. Additionally, air fryers promote portion control since most models have a limited capacity. Unlike giant oven interiors that encourage over-filling trays and mindless overeating, air fryer baskets help curb excess calorie intake. Air fryers also cook foods rapidly, which satisfies cravings fast before overeating occurs. For instance, you can make a batch of air fried fries in 12-15 minutes versus waiting 45 minutes or longer for oven-baked fries. For those prone to snacking between meals, having an air fryer on hand eliminates excuses that lead to grabbing unhealthy convenience snacks like chips, candy or fast food.

The ability to reheat leftovers is another air fryer feature that lends itself to weight loss success. Rather than ditching leftovers after a few days due to unappealing textures, the air fryer can revive them to taste freshly cooked. Reheating leftovers in the air fryer is quick and crisps them up nicely. This allows you to cook a few wholesome meals at the start of the week while still having tasty leftovers help avoid less healthy takeout options later on. The air fryer's reheating abilities help reduce food waste and eliminate the tendency to eat unplanned, impulsive meals.

In summary, integrating the air fryer into your regular meal preparation offers many benefits for pursuing overall healthy eating habits and managing your weight. It promotes convenience, allows you to adapt fried favorites into healthier versions, provides versatility beyond just air frying, enables creativity through diverse recipes, and supports portion and craving control—all of which are essential when trying to achieve a healthy lifestyle. With some basic tips and go-to recipes, the air fryer can transform into one of your kitchen's MVPs.

The Impact of the Air Fryer Diet on Weight Loss

When followed consistently, adopting an air fryer diet can have a profound impact on weight loss efforts. By utilizing the air fryer to prepare wholesome, low-fat meals, this diet provides an effective approach to reducing body fat and achieving a healthy weight.

Several key factors underpin just how an air fryer diet can ignite transformative weight loss. First and foremost, the air fryer significantly slashes the fat and calories in traditionally fried foods. By using rapid, superheated air instead of submerging foods in liters of oil, the air fryer reduces the fat and calorie load of recipes tremendously. Meals like fried chicken, french fries and onion rings can be enjoyed with just a teaspoon of oil rather than being drenched in grease.

Eliminating all that excess oil and fat is crucial for weight loss, as deep fried foods are extremely calorie dense. To illustrate, a serving of french fries cooked in a deep fryer contains over 500 calories and 30 grams of fat. The same portion air fried contains around 200 calories and 3 grams of fat. These major reductions in calories and fat quickly add up each day, creating the essential calorie deficit for weight loss.

Beyond frying with less oil, the air fryer diet emphasizes lean proteins like poultry, fish and eggs over fatty red meats. Fresh fruits and vegetables also take center stage, providing nutrients and fiber. Whole grains and legumes are complex carbs consumed in moderation, displacing refined carbs. These nutritious foods satisfy hunger while keeping portions and calories controlled. By filling up on lower calorie foods, it's easier to stay within daily caloric needs for weight loss.

The air fryer also makes sticking to this lower calorie diet much more sustainable in the long run. The appliance helps avoid the food boredom that often plagues diets, thanks to the wide variety of meals that can be cooked. From fajitas to falafel, the possibilities are endless. This versatility prevents feelings of deprivation that lead to diet derailment.

Furthermore, the satisfying recipes and properly portioned meals prevent hunger pangs, cravings, and binge eating which often sabotage weight loss efforts. Nutrient dense proteins and fiber filled veggies provide lasting fullness. Blood sugar and insulin levels remain steady thanks to low carb meals. These factors promote effective appetite control for consistent calorie restriction.

Several additional advantages of the air fryer diet facilitate fat burning and weight loss results. The focus on home cooked meals means less reliance on takeout, reducing exposure to excess calories, sodium and harmful fats. Air frying is fast and simple, making it more likely you will have time to prepare healthy meals versus grabbing fast food.

Above all, being able to still enjoy crispy, fried textures and richer flavors without all the fat and calories is very liberating psychologically. It reduces feelings of restriction and the urge to binge on greasy fare. The air fryer provides satisfaction and variety that makes sustaining the diet's calorie deficit easier over months and years.

Over time, sticking to this lower calorie air fryer diet by cooking flavorful, lean meals consistently creates a moderate daily calorie deficit. Experts recommend a deficit of 500-

750 calories per day for safe, sustainable weight loss. This normally results in losing 1-2 pounds per week on average, sometimes more in the beginning.

While the rate of loss may seem modest compared to extreme diets promising 10 pounds in a week, the air fryer diet leads to lasting results. Rapid initial weight loss is often just water weight that quickly returns. It also shocks your metabolism, causing rebound weight gain. Losing just 1-2 pounds of actual body fat weekly on the air fryer diet is reasonable and maintainable.

When combined with exercise, this steady fat loss adds up. Over 6 months, that could translate to over 50 pounds shed. The low carb focus also reduces muscle loss compared to more drastic calorie cuts. Preserving or building muscle helps maintain an active metabolism. The result is efficient, holistic body recomposition for improved health markers like cholesterol and blood pressure in addition to weight loss.

Scientific studies have validated the effectiveness of using an air fryer for weight control. One clinical trial compared weight loss and cardiometabolic risk factors on a low-fat air fryer diet versus counseling alone over 6 months. The air fryer group lost 4 times more weight than the counseling only group. They also showed greater reductions in body fat percentage, blood pressure and cholesterol.

Researchers concluded hot air frying provides similar results to other calorie controlled diets, with the added benefit of keeping total and saturated fat low while still providing the taste, texture and satisfaction of fried foods. This enhances long term compliance and weight maintenance. Other studies confirm that using an air fryer supports feelings of fullness and satisfaction compared to other low fat cooking methods.

While individual results may vary, the proven benefits of reduced calories, fat, and carbs coupled with satiating protein and fiber make the air fryer diet an evidence-backed strategy for weight loss. Some tips to maximize fat burning include pairing it with strength training to preserve metabolism-boosting muscle. Be sure to track macros and calories consistently, especially with high fat proteins and dressings. Weigh yourself weekly under the same conditions for an accurate gauge of progress.

Above all, consistency and patience are key to see enduring results. There will inevitably be plateaus and slow weeks, especially as you get closer to your goal weight and initial rapid water loss tapers off. Embracing the air fryer diet as a lifestyle, not a temporary fix, will pay dividends for your health and body over time. With commitment to the core principles, the pounds will continue to melt away.

So in summary, the air fryer diet absolutely can ignite amazing weight loss results. By drastically reducing the fat and calories in fried foods while preventing feelings of deprivation, it provides sustainable calorie control for safe fat burning. The focus on lean proteins, smart carbs and nutrient dense produce optimizes nutrition as well. When followed diligently for months and years, the pounds shed and health gains from an air fryer diet make it a truly transformative approach.

Preparing for Your Transformative Journey

Embarking on a weight loss journey is a major life change that requires commitment, preparation, and a positive mindset to set yourself up for success. While an air fryer opens up possibilities for healthy cooking, you must also do the mental and emotional groundwork to stay motivated. Preparing properly will help the air fryer diet lead to transformative results.

Start by re-examining your reasons for wanting to lose weight and improve your health. What exactly motivates you? Improved energy and mobility? Lowering health risks? Feeling confident and comfortable in your body again? Identify your "why" and refer back to it whenever you need inspiration.

Take an honest assessment of your current eating and activity habits without judgment. Where are there opportunities to incorporate more nutritious whole foods and enjoyable movement? Set SMART goals with specific action steps so you can track progress.

Assemble a support system of people who will cheer you on without judgement. Share your goals and journey with positive friends and family who will be in your corner through ups and downs. Their encouragement can make all the difference on tough days. Consider joining a support group or online community as well.

Educate yourself on smart low-carb eating and cooking techniques. Understanding nutrition fundamentals will empower you to make the best choices. Meal planning is also key—devote time each week to shop for healthy ingredients and batch prep recipes to set yourself up for success.

Clear out any highly processed temptations from your kitchen. Then restock your fridge and pantry with low-carb staples like vegetables, eggs, lean protein, healthy fats, and wholesome seasonings. Having the right foods on hand makes grabbing a nutritious meal or snack easy.

Schedule a physical exam and discuss your weight loss plans with your doctor, especially if you take medications that may require adjustment. Getting medically cleared shows you're taking your health seriously and gets you valuable support.

Make other lifestyle tweaks that facilitate healthy habits, like setting a bedtime that allows for adequate sleep. Add daily movement that you enjoy—this could be taking the stairs, walking with a friend, cycling, swimming. Anything that gets you moving matters!

Some find that journaling helps them stay accountable and notice healthy patterns emerging. Jot down meals, exercise, moods, and measurements. Over time, reflect on your entries to see the concrete impact your changes are having.

Be prepared for setbacks by making a plan for managing situations that may threaten your resolve. Identify your triggers—stress, certain social events, travel—and create strategies. If you slip up, get right back on track without letting it derail you.

Expect your tastes to change as your diet improves. You may discover new favorite foods. Keep trying new air fryer recipes until you have go-to meals that satisfy. Soon, wholesome eating will become habit.

Of course, transforming your lifestyle takes time. Make small, sustainable changes rather than extreme measures you can't maintain. Celebrate each little victory! Measure your progress in how you feel, not just the number on the scale.

The journey requires patience with yourself. If you have an off day, take it in stride and regroup. Focus on all the things you are doing right for your health rather than being perfect. Progress over perfection is the key.

Embark on your air fryer diet journey equipped with the tools, mindset and support you need to succeed. Approaching change thoughtfully and positively will serve you well on your path to improved health and wellbeing. Stay focused on your motivations and goals. Small steps will lead to big results over time. You've got this!

CHAPTER 2

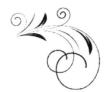

THE BASICS OF AIR FRYER COOKING

Getting to Know Your Air Fryer

P urchasing an air fryer opens up a world of quick, convenient and healthy cooking possibilities. However, as with any new kitchen gadget, there is a learning curve to fully master this versatile appliance. Taking the time to properly get acquainted with your air fryer will have you air frying like a pro in no time.

When unboxing your new air fryer, thoroughly read the included manual and product information to understand how to operate it safely. Air fryers come in several shapes and sizes, but they generally contain the same main components. These include a cooking basket, heating element, touch screen controls, and a crisping tray beneath the basket. Pay attention to accessories included, like recipe books and silicone tongs or grippers for handling the hot basket.

Once you've identified all the parts, wash the removable pieces in hot soapy water before using to remove any manufacturing residue. Double check that you've removed any protective plastic film or stickers from the touchscreen or other surfaces before powering the appliance on.

It's smart to run a test cycle while empty when using an air fryer for the first time. This preheats the appliance to burn off any lingering odors or chemicals from the manufacturing process. Set the temperature to 400°F for 3-5 minutes. You may notice some slight smoke or smells which is normal. Proceed to cook some basic foods while learning how your model works.

Start by air frying simple foods like frozen french fries, fresh vegetables tossed in oil or chicken pieces brushed with oil. Follow package instructions for optimal timing and temperature. Begin testing at the lowest suggested cooking time, checking food frequently until you understand your air fryer's timing tendencies. Unlike ovens, air fryers cook food much faster thanks to the concentrated heat circulation.

Pay attention to the sounds and airflow patterns from your air fryer's fan while cooking. Listen for any concerning noises like rattling, buzzing or grinding that could indicate an issue. Get accustomed to opening and closing the basket safely with the provided grippers and tongs. Always exercise caution when handling the extremely hot basket.

Once comfortable with the basics, consider doing a deep clean of the appliance. Over time, air fryers can accumulate grease residue or odors from cooking. Follow your model's cleaning instructions, usually either washing removable parts by hand or placing them in the dishwasher. For the interior, use a baking soda paste with a soft sponge or cloth to gently scrub away any debris.

After cleaning, break in the air fryer with flavorful foods that will leave a pleasant aroma inside, like baked cinnamon apples, citrus chicken or rosemary roasted potatoes. Pay attention to how full you pack the basket with different ingredients and whether they cook evenly. Part of getting acquainted with any air fryer is learning to arrange food in the optimal way for circulation.

For example, ingredients like fresh fries, chicken wings and nuggets may benefit from doing a mid-cook shake, pause or rearrange to promote browning. Vegetables and battered items may cook better in a single layer versus heaped piles. Take notes on cook times and settings with each trial recipe.

Once the basics are mastered, don't be afraid to push the limits of your air fryer's capabilities. Try out recipe ideas that utilize the air fryer's fan to dehydrate fruits, make beef jerky or dry herbs. Test reheating leftovers to restore crispy textures. Use it to quickly melt cheese atop nachos or crisp a pizza crust. Discover which foods cook best directly on the basket versus in a metal pan or silicone insert.

The key to unlocking the potential of your air fryer is being hands-on during the learning phase. Pay attention to inconsistencies or quirks specific to your appliance. Perhaps the fan seems weaker on one side, affecting even browning. If so, rotate your food midway through cooking. Get in the habit of gently shaking, tossing or flipping food for optimal texture and color.

In no time, you'll be able to operate your air fryer confidently without monitoring it constantly or relying on recipes. Though compact in size, these appliances perform a surprisingly wide array of cooking techniques. Frying, roasting, broiling, baking, dehydrating, reheating - an air fryer truly does it all in record time with minimal oil.

By taking the time upfront to understand your appliance's functions and nuances, you'll be able to masterfully prepare an array of delicious, healthful dishes. So embrace the learning curve and have fun unleashing the versatility of your air fryer. In no time, you'll be air frying everything under the sun to crispy, flavorful perfection.

Essential Tips for Air Fryer Beginners

Investing in an air fryer opens up a world of quick, convenient and healthy cooking options. Harnessing the power of superheated, rapidly circulating air, air fryers produce crispy "fried" foods, meat, vegetables and more using little to no oil. Like any new kitchen gadget, there is a learning curve to master air fryer cooking. Following some essential tips will help you get the most out of this versatile appliance as a beginner.

One of the top tips is to thoroughly read your model's manual so you understand how to operate and maintain it properly. While air fryers share common features and functions, each brand and model differs somewhat. Get acquainted with your machine's specific temperature and timer knobs, buttons or digital interfaces. Check that all parts and accessories listed are present, such as the fryer basket, drip tray, racks, etc. Familiarize yourself with the wattage, capacity and any special features like multiple rack levels or cooking pre-sets.

Before using most appliances, you would give them a test run but air fryers do not need "breaking in." You can start cooking right away once you understand the basic functions. That said, do remove all packing material and give the fryer basket and interior a wash beforehand. It's also smart to run the machine empty at 400 degrees for 4-5 minutes to burn off any manufacturing residue.

One rookie mistake is overcrowding the air fryer basket. Just like traditional frying, air flow is crucial! Overfilling prevents air from properly circulating and leads to uneven cooking. Get the best results by leaving at least a half inch space around foods. For larger items like chicken breasts, arrange them in a single layer without overlapping. You may have to cook in batches to avoid overcrowding. Use cooking spray or silicone liners to prevent sticking if needed.

While air fryers use little oil, a small amount of healthy cooking fat still goes a long way. Lightly brush or mist foods with olive, avocado or coconut oil before air frying. Oil helps facilitate even browning and makes the interior nicely moist. Spritzing veggies with lemon juice or vinegar also boosts caramelization. Dredging meat and veggies in a light mixture of oil and spices further enhances flavor.

Don't forget to preheat your air fryer before adding food. Air fryers cook very quickly once up to temperature. Preheating for 3-5 minutes allows the element and air to fully heat up so that food starts crisping immediately. Of course, adjust preheat timing based on the recipe and amount of food. For example, preheat 5 minutes for frozen foods but just 2-3 minutes for fresh.

While air fryers cook fast thanks to superhot air, food does need a little time for the heat to penetrate to the center and kill any bacteria. Meat especially requires thorough cooking for safety. That said, start checking food at the lower end of the recommended cook time range to avoid overcooking. You can always put it back in for a minute or two more if needed.

Use an instant read thermometer to accurately gauge doneness of proteins. Meat needs to reach safe internal temperatures to destroy bacteria and pathogens. Whole chicken should read 165°F, ground meats 160°F, steak/pork 145°F, and fish 140°F. The thermometer takes the guesswork out of determining doneness.

The air fryer makes cooking homemade fries and other potato dishes easy. Soak potato wedges, fries or cubes in cold water for 15 minutes before air frying to remove starch and prevent burning. Rinse then pat very dry before tossing with oil. Parcooking potatoes 5-7 minutes before air frying yields extra crispy results.

One advantage of the air fryer is being able to cook frozen foods with ease. There is no need to defrost beforehand. Simply add a few minutes to the cook time and adjust temperature as needed. Cooking spray prevents frozen items like fries or nuggets from sticking together. Air frying frozen foods makes speedy, healthy meals a breeze.

Take advantage of the air fryer's convection currents to cook multiple items with differing cook times together. Place delicate foods that require less time in the basket first, then add heartier items like meats. The superhot air will penetrate and cook everything through perfectly.

Foods that are battered or breaded like chicken tenders, fish sticks or jalapeno poppers turn out exceptionally crispy in the air fryer. Use lighter breadcrumb coatings rather than heavy beer batter for the best texture and crunch. Work in small batches to prevent crowding when frying breaded items.

One mistake to avoid is ignoring your air fryer's timer alerts. It will beep when done but food left sitting in the machine can overcook. Promptly remove items when finished cooking. Food retains heat and continues cooking slightly when removed from the hot air.

Take care not to overfill the fryer basket or overload its capacity. This varies by model but general guidance is 1-2 pounds of food per batch. Overloading prevents proper air circulation. If cooking large meals, work in smaller batches. Let the fryer fully reheat between batches for consistent results.

Patience is key when learning any new cooking method. It may take a few tries to master temperatures, cook times and how to arrange foods in your air fryer model. Refer to your manual's troubleshooting tips if needed. Varying factors like load size, food density, and even room temperature impact results. With practice, you will become an air frying expert!

In summary, reading your air fryer's manual, preheating properly, allowing airflow, using some oil, not overcrowding, checking for doneness and cooking in small batches sets you up for success as a beginner. Follow recipe directions and start checking for doneness at the lowest recommended cook times. Be patient – with use, you will get the hang of your machine for fantastic "fried" foods minus all the fat and grease!

Understanding Cooking Times and Temperatures

Mastering the ideal cooking times and temperatures is essential for air fryer success. With some basic knowledge and experimentation, you'll be able to achieve perfectly cooked results every time. Proper timing and temp control ensures your air fried foods turn out crispy, browned, and cooked through without burning or drying out.

As a general rule, air frying requires significantly less time than traditional frying or oven baking. The super hot, rapidly circulating air quickly crisps the exterior and cooks food from all sides simultaneously. Smaller items like chicken wings or vegetables may need only 10-15 minutes in the air fryer. Larger proteins like pork chops may require 15-20 minutes, and whole chickens 30-45 minutes depending on size.

These ranges are just a starting point though. The precise timing depends on several factors:

- Size and shape of food - Smaller items cook faster. Cut uniform sizes for even cooking.

- Amount of food - Don't overcrowd air fryer basket. Cook in smaller batches if needed.

- Type of food - Dense proteins take longer than tender vegetables. Moisture content impacts time.

- Preparation method - Breading, battering or saucing adds time. Frozen foods take longer.

- Personal taste - Adjust cook times up or down for desired doneness.

When trying a recipe for the first time, begin checking a few minutes early and extend time if needed. Let your eyes, nose and taste buds guide you. If an item isn't browning or crisping sufficiently, simply cook it longer.

For proteins like chicken, investing in an instant-read thermometer takes the guesswork out of determining doneness. But frequent peeking and nicking with a knife will also tell you when an item is cooked through.

To prevent overcooking, always immediately remove finished food rather than leaving it in heating up the air fryer. Items will continue cooking briefly after removed from the basket.

Air fryer temperature settings also impact cooking time. Most recipes call for cooking between 360-400°F, but you can adjust temperature up or down to achieve your desired texture and browning.

Lower temps around 300°F are ideal for gently cooking delicate fish or eggs without scorching the exterior. Higher temps up to 420°F will intensify browning and crisping, but risk burning food if you aren't diligent.

When air frying items with different cook times like vegetables and protein on the same sheet, set the temperature based on the item needing the highest temp. Then remove quicker cooking items as they finish.

You may need to turn or flip larger items midway through cooking to ensure even browning and heat penetration. But usually the super hot circulating air eliminates the need for flipping.

To prevent halting the cooking process and allowing heat to escape, resist opening the basket frequently. Use the air fryer window and built-in light to peek at progress.

While air fryer cooking times are typically shorter than oven baking, temperature guidelines are similar. Always refer to a recipe rather than guessing. As you become comfortable with your fryer you'll better understand exactly how long various foods should cook.

Keep notes in a cooking journal regarding what works for your particular model. Over time you will perfect the ideal air fryer times and temps to turn out mouthwatering meals. Don't be afraid to experiment until you find the formulas that work for your favorite foods.

With the right tools and a willingness to learn your appliance's nuances through trial and error, you will amaze yourself with how perfectly you can air fry everything from scratch-made chicken nuggets to crispy brussels sprouts to juicy pork tenderloin. Soon you'll be whipping up craveable meals for the whole family with ease.

Understanding the fundamentals of air fryer timing and temperature control is essential, but don't stress perfection. Allow yourself a learning curve as you grow comfortable with this new cooking technique and unlock all of its healthy possibilities.

Maintenance and Cleaning of Your Air Fryer

While air fryers simplify cooking with minimal oil, they still require regular maintenance and cleaning to function safely and effectively. Establishing good habits with your air fryer will extend its lifespan while preventing potential fires or malfunctions. Don't be intimidated—with just a few minutes after each use and occasional deep cleanings, keeping your air fryer pristine is easy.

The most vital habit is removing and safely discarding oil from the air fryer after each use. Even when cooking with little to no oil, residuals can accumulate in the bottom from food drippings. After the air fryer cools, remove the basket and dispense any excess oil from the reservoir at the bottom into a heat-safe container. Wipe the reservoir clean before replacing the basket. This simple ritual reduces the risk of grease buildup catching fire.

Additionally, always clean the air fryer basket and accessories promptly after cooking. Food debris left behind can burn onto the surfaces during subsequent cooking. Allow components to cool sufficiently after cooking, then wash with hot, soapy water. Use a soft brush or sponge to gently scrub away any stuck-on residue. Most air fryer baskets and pans feature nonstick coatings, so avoid abrasive scouring pads. If needed, fill the basket with water and dish soap, then run the air fryer for 5-10 minutes to loosen debris. Rinse and dry completely before next use.

For air fryer accessories like silicone molds or tongs, inspect manufacturer instructions before placing in the dishwasher. Hand washing is typically recommended. Pro tip: a dishwasher-safe silicone brush is perfect for scrubbing air fryer nooks and crannies.

While prompt cleaning prevents most buildup, oils and greases still accumulate over time, producing odors. Every few months, do a deep clean by removing all parts, including the heating coil guard. Check your manual for proper technique to avoid damaging components. Soak parts in hot, soapy water or a degreasing solution. Use a stiff nylon brush to scrub stubborn grease deposits before rinsing and drying fully.

Once disassembled, clean the interior with a baking soda and water paste and soft cloth, concentrating on vents and crevices near the heating element. Avoid submerging the electrical base in water or using metal scouring pads. Reassemble all components before use.

Maintaining your air fryer also means watching for signs of wear and damage. Inspect the power cord for fraying or cracks. Ensure the handle stays securely attached and components fit snugly together. If you notice rattling noises, strange smells or excess smoke, unplug the fryer and contact the manufacturer about potential issues or need for repairs.

With heavy use over time, the nonstick coating inside the cooking basket can deteriorate. Replacement air fryer baskets are available for purchase. Also consider replacing accessories like silicone molds, trays or protective inserts if they become warped, stained or damaged.

A well-cared-for air fryer should provide many years of use. Implementing a routine of quick cleanings after each meal and occasional deep cleanings keeps it looking and functioning like new. Here are some top tips for maintaining your air fryer:

- Discard oil and wipe basket after every use when cool

- Wash all parts with soap and water after each use

- Alternate cooking fatty and lean foods

- Deep clean unit every 2-3 months with degreaser

- Brush basket with oil before cooking for optimal nonstick effect

- Check for damage, odd noises or smells that could indicate issues

- Replace worn or damaged parts and accessories as needed

With regular easy cleanings and proper maintenance habits, your air fryer can continue cooking up quick, healthy and delicious meals safely and efficiently for years of enjoyment.

CHAPTER 3

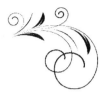

BREAKFAST RECIPES TO KICKSTART YOUR DAY

Low-Carb Air Fryer Breakfast Recipes

Starting your day with a wholesome, low-carb breakfast is one of the best ways to kickstart weight loss. The air fryer makes preparing delicious morning meals that align with your diet fast and easy. From omelets to avocado toast, read on for air fryer breakfast recipe ideas to break your fast in a slimming, yet satisfying way.

One of the most classic air fryer breakfasts is perfectly cooked eggs any style. The circulating hot air cooks eggs gently to your desired doneness, without drying them out or making them rubbery. To air fry eggs, simply spray the fryer basket with oil spray. Crack eggs directly into the basket holes to keep their shape intact. Air fry at 300°F for 3-5 minutes until eggs reach your desired consistency. Season with a pinch of salt and pepper. For an easy protein boost, add crumbled bacon or sausage along with veggies like onions, peppers or tomatoes.

Transform your eggs into fluffy omelets by whisking eggs thoroughly with a splash of milk or water before air frying. For a low-carb pizza omelet, top egg mixture with pepperoni, mushrooms, tomato sauce and mozzarella before air frying. Or make a veggie omelet with onions, peppers, spinach and feta. The possibilities are endless for customizable omelets.

Whip upperfect little egg bites in your air fryer for a grab-and-go breakfast. Grease a muffin tin and crack an egg into each crater, seasoning with salt and pepper. Add cheese, vegetables, meat or other mix-ins. Air fry at 300°F for 12-15 minutes until eggs are just set. Pop out the egg bites and store in the fridge or freezer.

One of the quickest air fryer breakfasts is avocado toast. Simply air fry bread in the basket until crisped on the edges while avoiding burning. Top toasted bread with mashed avocado and seasonings like red pepper flakes and lemon juice. For added nutrition, top with an egg made to your liking. You can even cook the egg right on top of the avocado toast!

Make jean-friendly sandwiches with air fried breakfast sausage patties or Canadian bacon medallions. Form sausage meat into patties and cook at 370°F for 8-10 minutes flipping halfway. For Canadian bacon, air fry thin slices for 4-5 minutes. These low-carb proteins pack a punch of savory flavor between bread or in a breakfast taco or burrito.

One of the most fun and family-friendly air fryer breakfasts is pancake or waffle "bowls." Mix up pancake batter, fill greased ramekins or waffle molds and air fry at 360°F for 7-9 minutes. Scoop out the cooked bowl and fill with yogurt and fruit for a perfectly portioned breakfast. For savory pancake bowls, add cooked sausage or bacon crumbles into the batter.

The air fryer also turns out picture-perfect stuffed breakfast pitas to power your morning. Fill halved pitas with whisked eggs, sautéed veggies and a sprinkle of cheese. Air fry at 325°F for 5-7 minutes until eggs are set. For a Mediterranean vibe, use feta, spinach and sundried tomatoes. Tex-Mex options include salsa, bell peppers and avocado.

Make pizza-stuffed breakfast calzones for a satisfying and portable morning meal. Roll out pizza dough into disks. Fill with scrambled eggs, cheese and other toppings like mushrooms, sausage or peppers. Fold dough over filling and seal edges. Air fry at 350°F for 6-8 minutes until golden brown. Let calzones cool slightly before digging in to avoid burning your mouth!

One of the simplest low-carb breakfasts is Greek yogurt sprinkled with berries, nuts and seeds. Air fried fruits like pineapple, peaches, apples or pears become sweet toppings too. To make your own low-sugar granola, toss rolled oats, nuts, coconut and spices in oil and air fry until toasted. Sprinkle this granola over yogurt for added crunch and flavor.

Banana oat muffins are another great on-the-go option. Mash ripe bananas with eggs, vanilla, oats and baking powder. For a nutty flavor, add chopped walnuts or pecans. Portion batter into greased or lined muffin cups. Air fry at 325°F for 12-14 minutes until a toothpick inserted comes out clean. These soft and moist muffins will satisfy your morning sweet tooth.

As you can see, the air fryer allows you to prepare a wide variety of delicious low-carb breakfasts in minutes. Wake up your morning routine with protein-packed eggs, savory meats, simple avo toast or even pancakes and muffins. With an air fryer, you can enjoy all your breakfast favorites guilt-free!

Quick and Easy Air Fryer Breakfast Ideas

Mornings often feel rushed and hectic. Making time for a nutritious breakfast may take a backseat to pressing tasks like getting the kids to school or prepping for work. But meal prepping simple, satisfying breakfasts in your air fryer ensures you start your day fueled for success rather than hungry and distracted.

The air fryer allows you to quickly cook breakfast favorites in a healthier way. By reducing excess oil, you can enjoy crispy bacon, fluffy frittatas, and perfectly baked breakfast sandwiches without sabotaging your goals.

Air frying also brings out delicious flavors and textures without needing to hover over a stovetop. Simply toss ingredients into the basket and let the air fryer work its magic while you get ready for your day.

Here are quick, easy breakfast recipes and ideas to add to your morning routine:

Banana Oatmeal - Toss old-fashioned oats with milk and mashed banana then air fry for creamy, caramelized oatmeal almost as fast as microwaving. Sweeten with a touch of honey or cinnamon if desired.

Sheet Pan Breakfast Hash - Load up a sheet pan with pre-cooked potatoes, vegetables like bell pepper and onion, and turkey sausage. Air fry until lightly crisped for a hearty protein-packed hash.

Southwestern Egg Muffins - Whip eggs with veggies, salsa and cotija cheese then pour into greased ramekins. Air fry for fluffy, grab-and-go egg bites.

Breakfast Sandwiches - Layer pre-cooked turkey sausage patties, egg and cheese between halves of an English muffin. Air fry wrapped in foil for melt-y sandwiches in minutes.

Chilaquiles - To crisp day-old tortilla chips, smother in enchilada sauce and cheese then air fry until melted and bubbly. Top with fried eggs for a quick Mexican breakfast.

Apple Fritters - Mix applesauce, vanilla and cinnamon into pancake batter. Fold in diced apples and air fry batter by tablespoonfuls into delicious fresh apple fritters.

Bacon and Eggs - Prepare bacon in the air fryer for crispy, fuss-free strips. Then bake eggs in ramekins at the same time for a classic combo in just minutes.

Breakfast Burritos - Wrap scrambled eggs, cheese, salsa and diced potatoes in a tortilla. Air fry the burritos seam-side down for an easy meal on the go.

Breakfast Pizza - Top a tortilla or pita with sausage gravy, scrambled eggs, bacon crumbles and cheese. Air fry for a hand-held savory breakfast pizza.

Yogurt Parfaits - Layer air fried fruit like peaches or berries with Greek yogurt and granola in a jar or glass for a grab-and-go morning treat.

Veggie Frittata - Whisk eggs with any diced veggies you have on hand. Pour into a greased cake pan and air fry until puffed and golden for sliceable egg pie.

Donuts - Roll store-bought biscuit dough in cinnamon sugar then air fry, flipping halfway for donuts in minutes. Dunk in coffee for a quick week-day treat!

With a little creativity and some easy batch-prep, your air fryer can revolutionize your morning routine. No longer will you need to sacrifice nutrition for precious time or resort to sugary cereals or drive-thrus.

Let your air fryer's efficient cooking take the pressure off so you can customize quick, wholesome breakfasts that fuel you through the day. Soon you'll wonder how you ever started mornings without it!

Tasty and Nutritious Egg Dishes

Thanks to their versatility, eggs are one of the most ubiquitous ingredients used in air frying. Beyond traditional fried eggs, the air fryer allows you to quickly prepare egg-based dishes from all over the globe. Explore new flavors and add nutrition to your diet through these diverse, mouthwatering egg recipes.

For a protein-packed start to the day, whip up the quintessential air fried egg. Simply spray the basket with oil, crack an egg directly in and air fry at 300°F for 4-5 minutes until the whites are set but yolks runny. Season with salt, pepper and fresh herbs. Make an egg sandwich by air frying an egg alongside Canadian bacon or sausage patties.

Frittatas are another excellent air fried breakfast. Whisk eggs with veggies, meat or cheese and pour into a greased ramekin or cake pan. Air fry at 350°F for 15-18 minutes until puffed and golden. Try variations like broccoli cheddar, sausage spinach or chili cheese frittatas. Portion and refrigerate leftovers for quick breakfasts all week.

For a grab-and-go morning meal, make egg muffins loaded with veggies and bacon or ham in silicone molds. Whisk eggs and milk together, stir in additions like onions, peppers, spinach and pre-cooked meat, then distribute between greased molds. Air fry at 300°F for 18-20 minutes until set. Freeze extras to reheat later.

The air fryer also shines for making eggs "baked" within vegetables. Pour whisked eggs over raw veggie slices like zucchini, tomato or potato arranged in the basket, then air fry until eggs firm up. Try new flavor combos like Eggs Provençal baked in tomato or Indian-style baked eggs with curry.

Quiches cooked in pie pans or silicone molds are simple yet impressive egg dishes for brunch. Blind bake a pie crust in the air fryer before filling with egg mixture and baking again until set. Experiment with fillings like bacon mushroom, broccoli cheddar or ham and Swiss. Serve slices warm or chilled.

For easy appetizers, make mini egg "muffins" by cracking an egg into muffin cups or silicone molds, seasoning the top, then air frying until the whites set. Try topping ideas like chives, crumbled bacon, salsa, shredded cheese or pesto.

Among the most universally loved egg recipes is the omelet, easily achieved in the air fryer. Pour egg mixture into a greased pan and air fry at 300°F for just 2-3 minutes until bubbling. Flip carefully with a spatula and cook another 1-2 minutes to set the underside. Keep omelet ingredients like cheese, spinach, ham or mushrooms on hand.

For a touch of Southwest flavor, whip up a breakfast burrito by combining scrambled eggs with salsa, black beans, peppers and cheese wrapped in a tortilla. Air fry at 370°F for 10 minutes until the burrito shell crisps.

Finally, explore sweet and savory Chinese egg custard options like steamed egg pudding or pan-fried egg tarts made in ramekins or silicone molds. The air fryer's circulating heat gently cooks the egg custard to silky perfection.

From grab-and-go breakfasts to impress-your-guests brunch dishes, eggs are endlessly versatile in the air fryer. They add protein, vitamins and minerals to your diet while keeping recipes simple, quick and healthy. With minimal prep and short cook times, the air fryer lets you enjoy an array of global egg specialties any time.

Healthy and Delicious Smoothies and Shakes

Smoothies and shakes make nutritious and delicious additions to the air fryer diet. Blending fruits, vegetables, protein powders and healthy fats creates guilt-free beverages perfect for breakfast, snacks or post-workout recovery. The air fryer even allows you to make crispy, protein-packed smoothie bowls. Read on for amazing smoothie and shake ideas to blend up on the air fryer diet.

Fruit smoothies provide an easy way to boost your produce intake. Berries, mangos, bananas and pineapples blend beautifully into sweet yet nourishing drinks. For green smoothies, leafy greens like spinach and kale pack a punch of antioxidants and magnesium. Cruciferous veggies like broccoli and cauliflower can also be blended in.

To avoid blood sugar spikes, balance fruits with healthy fats like avocado, nut butters or chia seeds and protein from Greek yogurt or collagen peptides. Cinnamon provides a hint of sweetness without added sugars. For an energizing boost, add coffee or matcha powder. Ice helps create a frosty, refreshing texture.

Some tasty fruit smoothie combinations include strawberry banana, peach mango and pineapple coconut. Get creative with your own fruity concoctions! For green smoothies, combine spinach, pineapple, banana, coconut water and lime. Or blend kale, mango, avocado and vanilla protein powder.

In addition to fruits and veggies, smoothies allow you to sneak extra protein into your diet. Whey, plant-based or collagen peptides dissolve seamlessly into smoothies, making them more satiating. Nut butters and Greek yogurt also provide sustaining protein and healthy fats.

For a nutty plant-based protein boost, blend silken tofu, peanut butter, cocoa powder, banana and almond milk. Or try a tropical post-workout recovery smoothie with pineapple, mango, vanilla whey and coconut water. There are endless smoothie possibilities to hit your protein needs!

Smoothies need not be limited to fruits and veggies. Unexpected ingredients like cauliflower, avocado and spinach make nutrient packed additions. Spices like cinnamon, nutmeg and ginger add flavor depth without calories.

Some unique combinations include almond butter, vanilla protein, cocoa powder, espresso and cauliflower for a frosty "milkshake." Blend avocado, Greek yogurt, matcha powder, spinach and mint for an earthy green treat. Let your imagination run wild!

Air fried fruits also make amazing smoothie boosters. Drizzle berries, peaches, bananas, pineapple and other fruits with cinnamon and air fry at 400°F for 5-8 minutes until softened. The caramelization enhances sweetness sans added sugar. Simply blend the air fried fruits with your other smoothie ingredients.

Beyond drinks, smoothies transition into healthy air fried breakfast bowls beautifully. Blend up your favorite fruits, proteins and veggies in the blender. Then pour the mixture into a greased ramekin and air fry at 400°F for 8-10 minutes until set.

Top with extra fruit, seeds, coconut flakes or granola for contrasting textures. You can also make chia pudding smoothie bowls by blending chia seeds, Greek yogurt and milk before air frying. The possibilities are endless for creative smoothie bowls!

In addition to smoothies, shakes make a slimming choice to satisfy sweet cravings on the air fryer diet. The air fryer allows you to whip up healthier versions of traditionally high-fat fast food shakes.

For a chocolate protein shake, blend cocoa powder, peanut butter, avocado and protein powder with your milk of choice. Air fry your own bananas before blending for extra sweetness. Or try this orange creamsicle shake: Blend fresh orange juice, vanilla Greek yogurt, vanilla protein powder and a pinch of orange zest.

Another slimming trick is turning your favorite smoothies into shake pops. Simply blend your smoothie, then pour into popsicle molds. Air fry at 275°F for 18-22 minutes, checking often, until pops are frozen through. Kids and adults alike will love these fun frozen treats!

Whipping up nutritious smoothies and shakes is effortless with the air fryer expanded arsenal of ingredients. Satisfy your sweet tooth while sneaking in extra protein, produce and healthy fats through these crave-worthy blended beverages.

Sweet Delights: Air Fryer Pastries and Pancakes

While a healthy air fryer diet mainly focuses on wholesome savory meals, there's definitely still room for the occasional sweet treat. Sinful deep-fried pastries and dripping-with-oil pancakes are out. But your air fryer lets you bake up lighter versions of classic breakfast indulgences and desserts by reducing excess oil and fat.

Making your own fresh pastries and pancakes is surprisingly easy with an air fryer. The hot air circulation gives them even browning and a deliciously crispy exterior while keeping the interior tender. Whip up these sweet delights on leisurely weekends for something special.

Fluffy Buttermilk Pancakes

You can easily make pancake batter from scratch in 5 minutes. Simply whisk together flour, baking powder, salt, sugar, milk, egg, and melted butter. For a wholesome tweak, replace some of the all-purpose flour with whole wheat flour and add a teaspoon of vanilla extract.

Lightly grease the air fryer basket with cooking spray or oil. Then pour in 2-3 tablespoonfuls of batter per pancake, leaving space between each. Air fry at 400F for 5-6 minutes until puffed and golden brown, flipping halfway.

Serve tall stacks of pancakes warm, topping with maple syrup, fresh fruit like berries or bananas, chopped nuts, lemon curd, mascarpone cheese, or other favorites for a special weekend treat.

Crispy French Toast

ForFrench toast, whisk together eggs, milk, cinnamon, vanilla and nutmeg. Quickly dip bread slices in the mixture, then air fry at 400F for 4-5 minutes per side until crispy outside and custardy inside.

Top with maple syrup, powdered sugar, sliced fruit, or even cream cheese icing if you want an extra decadent breakfast.

Flaky Cinnamon Rolls

Refrigerated canned biscuit dough makes cinnamon rolls a breeze. Simply flatten dough rounds, coat with melted butter, cinnamon and brown sugar, then tightly roll up.

Place sealed side down in the air fryer and cook at 350F for 12-15 minutes until puffed and golden.

Cream Cheese Danish

Flaky store-bought puff pastry can be transformed into sweet cheese danish treats.

Cut rectangles of puff pastry and sprinkle one half with cream cheese, powdered sugar, and lemon zest. Fold over other half and press edges to seal. Air fry for 8-10 minutes until golden brown.

Apple Hand Pies

Revisit the hand pies of your childhood, but in a healthier baked version. Thinly slice apples and mix with cinnamon, sugar, lemon juice and thickener like flour or cornstarch.

Spoon filling onto half of a flattened refrigerated pie crust round. Top with other half and crimp edges to seal. Cut slits in top. Air fry at 350F for 15 minutes until golden brown.

Mini Fruit Tarts

Press refrigerated sugar cookie dough into mini tart pans and air fry at 350F for 5-7 minutes until set. Let cool then top with fresh fruit, lemon curd, pastry cream or whipped cream for petite fruit tarts.

Molten Lava Cakes

For an indulgent chocolate dessert, make individual molten lava cakes.

Mix chocolate chips, butter, sugar, flour and eggs until smooth. Pour batter into greased ramekins and air fry for 8-10 minutes at 350F. The outside will cook while the inside stays gooey.

Satisfy your sweet tooth with air fried pastries and pancakes that cut fat and calories without sacrificing taste. Whip up a batch on lazy weekends for special family breakfasts or desserts.

CHAPTER 4

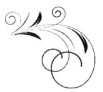

LUNCH AND DINNER RECIPES FOR BALANCED NUTRITION

Satisfying Air Fryer Chicken Recipes

From juicy boneless chicken breasts to crispy wings and tenders, air fried chicken is a lean protein staple perfect for any meal. The air fryer's rapid circulating heat locks in moisture while crisping up the exterior to perfection. Explore endless flavorful and satisfying chicken recipes made easy in the air fryer.

For weeknight meals, air fry bone-in chicken pieces like breasts, thighs or drumsticks coated in breadcrumbs or seasoned flour. The air fryer's concentrated heat thoroughly cooks chicken while browning the exterior. boneless chicken breasts also cook quickly from frozen. Pound them to even thickness and brush with oil and seasoning before air frying.

Give chicken wings and drumettes irresistible crispy exteriors without the oil of deep frying. Toss wings in cornstarch, potato starch or baking powder before air frying to achieve maximum crispiness. The small basket size of air fryers is perfect for cooking wings in even batches.

Chicken tenders are ideal for air frying whether homemade or frozen. Coat in breadcrumbs, panko or flour seasoned with onion powder, paprika, garlic powder and salt. Air fry in a single layer at 400°F for 8-10 minutes until browned and cooked through. Flip halfway for even browning.

For juicy roasted whole chickens, season a 4-5 pound bird inside and out then place breast-side down in the air fryer basket. Air fry at 350°F for 50-60 minutes until the thighs reach 165°F. Let rest before carving. The skin crisps up perfectly without needing to flip.

Give chicken vegetable stir fries an easy makeover by swapping out wok cooking. Cut raw chicken and veggies into small uniform pieces. Toss with cornstarch, oil and sauce ingredients. Air fry in a single layer, stirring occasionally, until chicken is cooked through and veggies tender-crisp.

Chicken also pairs well with cheese and sauces in the air fryer. Make chicken parmesan from frozen chicken breasts, tomato sauce and mozzarella. Use mayo, mustard or yogurt-based marinades to keep lean chicken breasts extra juicy.

For a Mexican-inspired dinner, coat chicken pieces with chili powder, cumin and garlic before air frying. Serve topped with fresh pico de gallo, avocado and cotija cheese. Or make crispy tacos with diced air fried chicken tossed with onions, peppers and seasoning folded into warmed corn tortillas.

Give chicken sandwiches and wraps next-level flavor straight from the air fryer. Cook boneless thighs or breasts until nearly done then quickly melt cheese on top while still in the basket. For crispy chicken wraps, coat chicken strips with seasoned flour and air fry until golden brown then wrap in flatbread with veggies and ranch dressing.

The air fryer can even handle moist, delicious chicken casseroles and pasta dishes. Combine diced chicken with sauce, pasta, rice or veggies in a baking dish then air fry until bubbling and cooked through. Try chicken alfredo, chicken & broccoli casserole or chicken fried rice.

With the speed and convenience of the air fryer, flavorful chicken dinners can be on the table any night of the week. The concentrated heat helps chicken of all cuts and types achieve a tender interior with an irresistibly crispy browned crust. Keep your chicken recipes exciting by exploring globally inspired seasonings and sauce options.

Hearty Beef and Pork Dishes

While chicken and fish feature heavily in the air fryer diet, occasional moderate portions of lean beef and pork provide variety and robust flavor. Their savory umami quality satisfies comfort food cravings in a healthier way. This chapter will explore juicy steaks, succulent roasts, zesty tacos and more air fryer beef and pork recipe ideas.

Sirloin, flank, chuck eye or tri-tip steaks cook quickly to juicy doneness in the air fryer without the hassle of grilling. Pat steaks dry and season generously with salt, pepper and spices like garlic powder or paprika. Let rest 15-30 minutes to absorb flavors. Air fry at 400°F for 4-8 minutes per side based on thickness. Use an instant read thermometer to test for your desired doneness, usually between 145-165°F. Rest steaks 5 minutes before slicing against the grain. Pair with roasted veggies for a satisfying meal.

Transform a steak into a hearty Philly cheesesteak sandwich by topping with sautéed onions, peppers and melted cheese on a crisp hoagie bun. Adding grilled mushrooms or a slice of air fried egg takes it over the top. You can even chop up leftover steak to make cheesy steak nachos in the air fryer.

Quick-cook cubed steak or chicken fried steak turn out remarkably crispy and tender in the air fryer without requiring deep frying. Pound steaks thin and dredge in an egg wash followed by seasoned flour or panko breadcrumbs. Mist with oil spray and air fry at 390°F for 7-9 minutes per side. Pair with mashed cauliflower or roasted potatoes to soak up the delicious gravy.

Roasts and larger cuts like brisket, tri-tip and chuck roast require more time to become fork-tender but the air fryer still cooks them 40-50% faster than traditional ovens with fantastic results. Season roasts all over and cook at 325°F until meat reaches 185-210°F internally. Baste occasionally with pan juices for added moisture and savor.

Perfectly cooked pork chops and boneless loin roast also shine via air frying. The circulating hot air seals in juices while creating a beautiful brown exterior crust on chops and roasts. Brine lean chops for added moistness before air frying with a spice rub.

While beef and pork are higher fat meats, proper air fryer cooking prevents excess grease for a leaner finished dish. Invest in a basket and pans that allow fats to drain away while food air fries. Clean the air fryer and empty the grease receptacle frequently to prevent buildup.

In addition to enjoying pork and beef on their own, they make amazing additions to lively tacos, burritos, fajitas, wraps, flatbreads and more. Flank steak fajitas sizzle with peppers and onions. Pulled pork or black bean tacos satisfy on homemade corn tortillas. The options for global flavor combinations are endless!

Lean ground beef or turkey cooked in the air fryer makes better-for-you meatballs, burgers, meatloaf and stuffed peppers. For turkey or beef meatballs, combine ground meat with breadcrumbs, egg, minced onions and seasoning. Roll into balls and mist with avocado oil spray. Air fry at 400°F for 8-10 minutes. Toss with low-carb marinara sauce and serve over zucchini noodles. Yum!

To air fry burgers, form patties slightly wider than your burger bun as meat shrinks. Place patties in the air fryer basket without stacking or crowding. Cook at 390°F for 6-10 minutes flipped halfway depending on thickness. Melting cheese on burgers the last 1-2 minutes keeps it crispy. Serve on lettuce wrapped buns with all the fixings.

Stuffed peppers also make for a fun and family-friendly air fried meal. Fill bell pepper halves with a mixture of cooked ground meat, riced cauliflower, tomato sauce and shredded cheese. Air fry at 350°F for 10 minutes until peppers soften adding a couple minutes for fully cooked fillings.

The variety of globally inspired beef and pork dishes you can make in the air fryer is endless. Consider easy Korean lettuce wraps, Greek pork souvlaki or empanadas. With scrumptious options from all corners of the world, your family and tastebuds will never tire of air fried beef and pork meals in healthy moderation.

Delicious and Nutritious Seafood Recipes

Seafood is a lean, protein-packed addition to any healthy diet. Fish and shellfish provide important omega-3 fatty acids and are relatively low in calories compared to other proteins. The air fryer lets you cook seafood to crispy, juicy perfection without needing to fuss with oil or constant watch. Enjoy your favorites guilt-free with these tasty recipes.

Crispy Fish Sticks

Cut wild caught white fish like tilapia or cod into long strips for homemade fish sticks. Toss with a little cornstarch and seasoning. Mist fish with oil then air fry at 400F for 5-6 minutes until browned, flipping halfway. Serve with spicy mayo or tartar sauce for dipping.

Coconut Shrimp

Butterfly peeled raw shrimp by slicing almost through the top. Skewer flat shrimp onto pre-soaked bamboo sticks. Dip in egg, then shredded coconut seasoned with sesame oil, salt and red pepper flakes. Air fry at 400F for 5-7 minutes until coconut is toasted.

Crab Cakes

Mix together cooked fresh or canned crabmeat, breadcrumbs, egg, lemon zest, Worcestershire sauce, Dijon mustard, scallions, and spices. Shape into patties and mist tops with oil. Air fry at 400F for 10-12 minutes, gently flipping halfway until golden brown.

Baked Lobster Tails

Thaw frozen lobster tails and use kitchen shears to cut through the top of the shell down the length of the tail. Brush with olive oil and seasonings. Air fry at 350F for 9-11 minutes until opaque. Drizzle with butter.

Blackened Salmon

Coat salmon fillets with Cajun seasoning and quick-mix blackening spice blend. Lightly mist fillets with avocado oil spray then air fry at 400F for 10-12 minutes until cooked through and flakes easily with a fork.

Breaded Scallops

Toss sea scallops in seasoned flour then egg wash then panko breadcrumbs. Mist the breaded scallops with oil and air fry at 400F for 7-9 minutes, gently turning halfway, until browned and cooked through.

Garlic Shrimp Skewers

Thread peeled raw shrimp onto skewers alternating with cherry tomatoes and chunks of lemon. Sprinkle with minced garlic, Italian seasoning, salt and pepper. Lightly drizzle shrimp with olive oil and air fry at 380F for 5-7 minutes until cooked through, turning skewers halfway.

Sweet Chili Salmon

Make crispy salmon poppers in your air fryer by brushing salmon slices with Asian sweet chili sauce then coating in panko crumbs. Air fry at 400F for 6-8 minutes until flaky, turning halfway.

With your air fryer, you can whip up succulent seafood entrees and appetizers that keep calories and fat in check while pumping up nutrition. Explore healthy preparations to find new favorites, like baked fish tacos, coconut crusted shrimp, or scallops with risotto and veggies.

Vegetarian and Vegan Options

One of the air fryer's strengths is its ability to create delicious vegetarian and vegan dishes. The circulating hot air crisps up veggies, tofu, tempeh and more with recipes that even meat lovers will enjoy. Explore the versatility of the air fryer to make any meal meatless.

For breakfast, air fry up veggie-packed scrambles and frittatas. Dice and air fry potatoes first before adding whisked eggs and veggies like spinach, peppers and onions. For vegan frittatas, blend tofu with nutritional yeast, veggies and seasonings before air frying. Make satisfying veggie omelets or burritos filled with air fried potatoes, peppers, beans, and avocado.

Snack on crispy air fried veggie chips like sweet potato, beet, or zucchini slices for a nutritious alternative to greasy potato chips. Season with spices like chili powder, garlic powder or cumin before air frying. Make batches to grab for a quick snack any time. Serve with hummus or guacamole.

One of the easiest ways to air fry vegetarian meals is roasting vegetables. Cubed root veggies like potatoes, sweet potatoes, and beets become caramelized and tender. Toss brussels sprouts or broccoli florets with oil and seasonings for an easy side. Though quick, air fried vegetables taste roasted!

Take vegetables up a notch with batters and breadings. Try air fried avocado fries, eggplant cutlets, or cauliflower "wings" and "steaks" breaded with panko, cornflakes or gluten-free crumbs. The air fryer makes veggie fritters, falafel and tempura come out perfectly crispy.

For hearty vegetarian mains, marinated tofu and tempeh become crispy and full of flavor when air fried. Press water out of tofu before marinating in sauces like Korean barbecue, teriyaki, or spicy buffalo style. Cut tempeh into strips and air fry with seasonings like garlic, paprika and cumin. For extra crunch, coat tofu and tempeh in cornmeal or panko before frying.

Turn extra firm tofu into versatile air fried "meats" for vegan dishes. Slice it into cutlets, dice it for stir-fries or crumble for tacos. To make vegan orange chicken, coat diced tofu in orange marmalade mixed with rice vinegar, soy sauce, garlic and chili flakes before air frying until caramelized.

Whip up vegetable fritters, falafel and faux meat croquettes from bean and grain mixtures formed into patties or balls. Try combinations like brown rice, mushrooms and walnuts for a hearty texture. Air fry in batches at 360 F until browned and crisp.

For a quick plant-based dinner, top a baked potato, sweet potato or squash with chili, tacos or a vegan shepherd's pie filling loaded with veggies like corn, peas, carrots and onion. Bake the potatoes first in the air fryer before splitting and stuffing.

Even classic comfort foods can be made vegetarian in the air fryer. Swap out pepperoni for mushrooms on air fried pizza and load vegetable casseroles like eggplant parmesan into ramekins before air frying until bubbly. Cook mac and cheese with broccoli, cauliflower or butternut squash mixed into the sauce.

Prepare nearly any vegetable perfectly in the air fryer. The concentrated heat browns and crisps while locking in moisture, unlike oven cooking which can dry out veggies. Always toss vegetables in a small amount of oil before seasoning and air frying for a delicious caramelized result.

With a plethora of possibilities, eating more vegetables has never been easier or more appetizing. The air fryer allows you to re-imagine typically meat-centric dishes into vegetarian delights through the power of crisp, robust flavors.

Quick and Easy Side Dishes

The best part of cooking main dishes in the air fryer is that you can make slimming sides at the same time with little extra effort. Round out your plate with nutritious vegetables, whole grains, legumes and more cooked conveniently and deliciously in your air fryer. This chapter will explore diverse recipe ideas for effortless appetizers, vegetables, beans, grains and other sides to complete balanced meals.

Appetizer-style sides like wings, chips and poppers are air fryer staples that make fun additions to meals in moderation. Toss chicken wings or drumettes in tangy Buffalo sauce post air frying for a spicy kick. For guilt-free chips, slice potatoes, parsnips, or jicama paper thin and air fry with seasoning until crispy. Or stuff sliced jalapeños with cheese before air frying for creamy, spicy poppers.

Roasting is one of the most popular uses for the air fryer as the superheated air circulates around vegetables, evenly caramelizing their natural sugars. First prep veggies by cutting larger pieces into bite-sized chunks and leaving petite vegetables whole. Toss chunks with just a little oil or mist with spray before air frying.

Root vegetables like potatoes, sweet potatoes, carrots and parsnips develop an amazing crisp exterior while turning tender inside when air fried. Brushing with oil and spices like garlic powder, paprika, or cumin kicks up the flavor.

Cruciferous vegetables also shine when air fried. Try cauliflower florets seasoned with curry powder or turmeric for an Indian twist. Air fry Brussels sprouts halved or quartered with olive oil, salt and pepper. Even a whole head of broccoli or Romanesco comes out perfectly caramelized and crisp-tender.

Beyond roots and crucifers, asparagus, peppers, zucchini, green beans and okra all cook up crispy and delicious with just a quick mist of oil. For ultimate flavor, toss veggies with minced garlic, citrus juice and zest, Parmesan cheese or fresh herbs before air frying.

Don't stop at just "roasting" veggies in the air fryer though – there are so many possibilities to try! Make veggie fries by cutting potatoes, carrots, beets or zucchini into matchsticks. Bread veggies for irresistible bites like fried zucchini sticks, eggplant chips or buttermilk okra. The options are limitless.

Whole grains like quinoa, farro, brown rice and bulgur provide satisfying complex carbohydrates as side dishes. Rinsing grains before cooking removes excess starch for fluffier results. The air fryer makes grains hands-off – just add to a baking pan with water or broth and cook at 350°F until tender.

For easy weeknight sides, cook quick-cooking grains like couscous, quinoa or bulgur right in the air fryer. Start with a 1 to 2 parts liquid to grain ratio and adjust moisture as needed. Allow extra time for larger grains like farro or wheat berries. Toss cooked grains with herbs, nuts or dressing for flavor.

In addition to grains, beans and legumes like chickpeas, black beans and lentils work wonderfully as plant-based protein sides. Cover dried beans with water and cook low and slow in the air fryer at 275-300°F until tender, 2-4 hours. Flavor beans with spices during or top prepared beans with sauces.

Canned beans need only a quick crisping in the air fryer. Rinse and drain beans then pat very dry before misting with oil. Air fry at 400°F for 6-8 minutes, shaking once. Season to taste – Mexican flavors like cumin, chili powder and lime work well. Or toss white beans with garlic and rosemary.

Don't limit yourself to traditional pairings either. Unexpected combinations like air fried Brussels and beans, sweet potatoes stuffed with farro or quinoa fried "rice" with riced broccoli keep mealtime exciting. Use your creativity and the possibilities are endless for slimming air fryer sides.

CHAPTER 5

SNACKS AND APPETIZERS FOR EVERY OCCASION

Low-Carb Air Fryer Snacks

Snacking can be an enjoyable part of any healthy eating plan as long as you choose the right options. When an afternoon craving strikes, resist the urge for crackers, chips, or other starchy offerings. With a little creativity, your air fryer can turn out crave-worthy low-carb snacks that satisfy with more nutrition and less guilt.

One of the easiest swap-outs is replacing potato chips or cheese crackers with snackable veggies. Air frying crisps vegetables without loads of added oil for crunch and flavor.

Baked Zucchini Chips - Toss thin slices of zucchini in garlic powder, salt, pepper and a spritz of oil. Air fry at 400F for 5-7 minutes until browned and crispy.

Beet Chips - Peel and thinly slice beets. Toss with avocado oil, salt and pepper. Air fry at 400F for 12-15 minutes, tossing halfway until dehydrated and crispy.

Kale Chips - Remove kale ribs and tear into pieces. Toss with oil, vinegar and seasoning. Air fry at 300F for 12-15 minutes until perfectly crisped.

Spicy Roasted Chickpeas - Drain and rinse canned chickpeas. Toss with olive oil, cumin, chili powder and a pinch of cayenne. Air fry at 400F for 15-20 minutes until browned and crunchy.

You can also transform proteins like deli meats and cheeses into quick, filling low-carb snacks.

Pizza Parcels - Wrap sliced pepperoni and mozzarella cheese in circles of pepperoni. Air fry for 5-7 minutes at 350F until the cheese melts.

Cheesy Bacon Crisps - Weave bacon slices into bundles then wrap cheese cubes inside. Air fry at 400F for 4-5 minutes until the bacon crisps.

Baked Cheese Bites - Press shredded cheeses like cheddar, Swiss or mozzarella into mini muffin tins. Air fry at 350F for 5-7 minutes until melted.

Pepperoni Chips - Arrange slices of pepperoni in a single layer on a parchment lined pan. Air fry at 400F for 5-7 minutes until crispy.

Get creative with other proteins like chicken, eggs and fish for tempting low-carb snacks straight from your air fryer.

Sesame Chicken Bites - Toss cubed chicken breast in soy sauce, honey, and sesame seeds. Air fry at 400F for 8-10 minutes until cooked through and glazed.

Deviled Eggs - Air fry hard-boiled eggs. Halve and scoop yolks into a bowl, mash with mayo, mustard and seasoning, then spoon back into whites.

Salmon Cakes - Mix canned salmon with breadcrumbs, egg, herbs and spices. Scoop into mini-patties and air fry at 400F for 5-7 minutes until browned and flaky.

Crunchy, savory snacks straight from your air fryer will squash cravings and energize your day without derailing your goals. Get creative with proteins, vegetables and healthy fats for quick bites packed with nutrition.

Perfectly-Crisped Vegetable Snacks

Crispy, crunchy vegetable chips and snacks are a nutritious way to cure cravings and bridge meals. The air fryer's rapid air circulation transforms fresh veggies into crave-worthy crisps and fries without deep frying. Explore the limitless potential for creating homemade vegetable snacks packed with flavor.

For classic potato fries with a lighter twist, the air fryer can't be beat. Cut potatoes into 1/4 to 1/2-inch fries, soak in cold water for 30 minutes to remove starch, then pat very dry. Toss with a tablespoon of oil and air fry at 400°F in a single layer for 12-15 minutes, shaking halfway. Sprinkle with salt and dip in your favorite condiment.

Sweet potatoes also make delectable oven fries. The natural sugars caramelize in the air fryer for irresistible sweet potato fries. Cut them a bit thicker than russet potatoes since they cook faster. Follow the same method as regular fries, reducing time to 10-12 minutes.

Veggies like carrots, parsnips, and beets transform into irresistible fries with the air fryer's concentrated heat. Peel vegetables if preferred, then cut into evenly-sized fry shapes. Toss with just a drizzle of oil, season with spices like chili powder or cumin, and air fry until tender-crisp.

For alternative veggie "chip" snacks, select produce with enough natural moisture like zucchini, eggplant or jicama. Slice thinly into rounds or sticks, sprinkle with salt and pepper, and air fry at 375°F for 5-8 minutes until crispy edges form.

Cabbage leaves also become marvelously crispy chips after air frying. Separate leaves from the core, brush lightly with oil and air fry at 350°F for 4-6 minutes until edges brown. Season with paprika, ranch powder or parmesan.

Make beet chips by trimming beetroots and slicing paper thin using a mandolin. Toss slices with oil and citrus zest before air frying at 350°F until dehydrated and crispy.

Even lettuce and greens turn into crispy baked snacks. Separate leaves, drizzle with oil and air fry at 300°F for 4-5 minutes. Kale chips become addictively crunchy thanks to the air fryer's circulation and concentrated heat.

For pungent vegetable crisps, slice radishes or Brussels sprouts very thinly. Toss with oil, salt and pepper and air fry at 375°F, shaking halfway until browned and dried.

Nearly any vegetable transforms from crispy snacks in the air fryer. Try carrot sticks, broccoli florets, cauliflower, snap peas, asparagus or bell peppers prepared the same way. Adjust temperature and time as needed to reach desired texture without burning.

Not limited to savory, air fried fruit chips make a sweet and healthy alternative to cookies or candy. Thinly slice apples, peaches, pears, pineapple or mango and air fry with a sprinkle of cinnamon. Banana chips are also delicious dehydrated in the air fryer with just a mist of oil to prevent sticking.

For ultimate customization, make your own veggie or fruit chip seasoning mixes to use. Combine salts with spices like chili powder, garlic powder, onion powder, smoked paprika or cumin. Dehydrated veggie powders like tomato, carrot or beet make colorful seasoning accents.

The air fryer allows you to turn farmers market finds into addictive crispy snacks bursting with nutrients. Follow basic slicing, oiling and air frying methods while exploring creative seasoning combinations. Keep bags of your homemade veggie and fruit chips on hand for wholesome snacking any time.

Air Fryer Finger Foods for Parties

Hosting a party or game day get-together? The air fryer allows you to cook up a spread of flavorful finger foods and appetizers that will wow your guests. Ditch the greasy fried fare in favor of these slimming yet totally satisfying party bites made efficiently in the air fryer.

Classic fried starters like wings, chicken nuggets and cheese sticks become lighter yet crispy bites with the air fryer's help. Mist raw wings with oil and cook at 400°F for 15-20 minutes until browned and cooked through, shaking occasionally.

Homemade baked chicken or turkey tenders and nuggets also cook up perfectly with just a light breadcrumb coating. Try lighter coatings like panko breadcrumbs, almond flour or pork rind crumbs. Pair wings and nuggets with carrot and celery sticks plus healthier dips like hummus or Greek yogurt ranch.

For crispy cheese sticks, coat mozzarella sticks with egg and Italian seasoned panko crumbs. Air fry at 400°F for 5-6 minutes flipping over halfway through. Serve with warm marinara sauce for dipping.

In addition to fried favorites, the air fryer lets you craft creative hot finger foods featuring vegetables, lean meats and more. Try these fun party appetizer ideas:

- Veggie spring rolls stuffed with shredded carrots, cabbage, bell peppers, mushrooms and water chestnuts tightly wrapped in rice paper and air fried until crispy.

- Mini bell pepper "pizzas" topped with sauce, veggies and a sprinkle of cheese then air fried until melty.

- Meatballs made from chicken, turkey, or lean beef simmered in tomato sauce after air frying. Offer toothpicks for easy picking.

- Crispy zucchini fries or sticks coated in Parmesan cheese, panko and spices before being air fried.

- Veggie-packed samosas with your favorite seasoned potato and pea filling wrapped in dough triangles then baked.

- Spinach and artichoke dip served warm and bubbly in a mini baked potato or mushroom cap "bowl".

- Maple bacon wrapped sweet potato fries for a hint of salty-sweet flavor.

- Falafel fritters made from chickpeas and seasoned vegan-friendly then air fried until crisp on the outside.

- Crispy cauliflower "wings" tossed in Buffalo sauce after air frying for a slimmer twist.

- Bite-sized eggplant or chickpea panisse fries perfect for dunking in creamy sauces.

The possibilities are endless for unique vegetarian and vegan-friendly air fried appetizers. Meat eaters will devour mini bacon wrapped sausages, crispy Korean chicken skewers or crunchy pork wontons too.

To make appetizers more portable for mingling guests, serve bite-sized foods in mini muffin tins, bamboo boats or on toothpicks or skewers. Offer a selection of dips like guacamole, salsa, hummus and tzatziki to round out your finger food spread.

Clean-up is easy when cooking in batches in the air fryer. Preheat for a few minutes between batches to maintain crispness. Keep air fried foods warm in a 200°F oven while cooking the rest.

To keep prep work manageable when expecting a crowd, take advantage of make-ahead options. Many appetizers can be partially or fully prepared then finished cooking just before serving.

So swap out greasy fried snacks in favor of lighter yet irresistible air fried finger foods. With the air fryer's help, you can be the host with the most appetizing spread without the extra fat and calories!

Healthy and Tasty Dips and Spreads

Dips and spreads are popular for snacking and appetizers, but many are laden with excess fat, salt, and calories. With your air fryer, you can transform wholesome ingredients into homemade dips and spreads that taste decadent yet nourish your body.

Whipping up your own fresh dips allows you to control what goes in them. Opt for Greek yogurt over sour cream, use reduced-fat cheeses, and load up on veggies to lighten traditional recipes. Air frying intensify flavors and textures without needing to fry in copious oil.

Roasted Red Pepper Dip

Char fresh red peppers under the air fryer broiler setting or on the stovetop. Place in a covered bowl to steam, then peel off the skins. Purée peppers in a food processor with feta, garlic, olive oil, and herbs. Air fry pita chips to dip.

Artichoke Spinach Dip

Drain and chop marinated artichoke hearts and mix together with thawed chopped spinach, grated Parmesan, Greek yogurt, garlic, and seasonings. Transfer to a baking dish and air fry at 400F for 10-12 minutes until heated through and browned on top. Serve with celery sticks or zucchini rounds.

Warm Crab Dip

Blend together crab meat, cream cheese, sour cream, lemon juice, Worcestershire sauce, Old Bay seasoning, and scallions. Transfer to a baking dish and air fry at 350F for 10-12 minutes until warmed through and bubbly on top. Serve with crackers or raw veggies.

Chickpea Hummus

Purée canned chickpeas, tahini, olive oil, garlic, lemon juice, and seasonings in a food processor until smooth. Transfer to a shallow baking dish and air fry at 400F for 6-8 minutes until heated through. Drizzle with olive oil and paprika. Enjoy with fresh vegetable crudités.

Queso Fundido

Mix together Monterey Jack and Oaxaca cheeses with crumbled chorizo. Transfer to a greased baking dish and top with pickled jalapeños. Air fry at 350F for 6-8 minutes until melted and bubbly. Serve with tortilla chips.

Homemade Salsa

Chop tomatoes, onions, jalapeño, cilantro and lime juice. Spread in an even layer on a parchment lined pan. Air fry at 400F for 10-12 minutes, stirring occasionally, until slightly dehydrated. Add salt and pepper. Enjoy with low-carb snacks.

Fresh Fruit Spread

Purée your favorite fruits like mango, strawberry, peach, or apricot in a blender until smooth. Spread into a parchment-lined air fryer basket in an even 1/4-inch layer. Air fry at 300F for 60-90 minutes, stirring every 20 minutes, until thickened to a jam consistency.

Whipping up homemade dips, spreads and salsas allows you to control the quality of ingredients. The air fryer helps intensify flavors for delicious appetizers and snacks that align with your healthy goals. Get creative with different herb and spice blends or mix-ins like roasted vegetables, beans, cheeses and fresh herbs.

CHAPTER 6

DELECTABLE DESSERTS FOR THE SWEET TOOTH

Guilt-Free Air Fryer Desserts

One of the biggest appeals of the air fryer is its ability to create healthier versions of traditionally sinful fried treats. With circulating hot air instead of greasy oil, you can indulge your sweet tooth with less guilt. Discover how simple desserts get magically transformed when air fried.

Air fried donuts prove you can teach an old dog new tricks. Prepare easy donut batter or pick up ready-made balls from the store. Air fry oiled donuts at 400F for 4-5 minutes until golden brown, flipping halfway. Coat in cinnamon sugar while warm!

Churros become delightfully crispy with only a fraction of the oil of conventional frying. Pipe eclair-like dough into the air fryer, air fry at 400F for 5-7 minutes flipping once, then roll in cinnamon sugar.

Fried pies like apple, cherry, or peach transform when air fried. Prepare double crust pies, vent steam holes, then air fry at 350F for 12-14 minutes until golden. Brush crust lightly with oil or butter for crisping.

Almost any baked goods come out perfectly in the air fryer through its precise temperature circulation. Make cookies, scones, muffins or biscuits for a quick batch with no preheating.

For single-serving brownies and blondies, pour batter into a ramekin, silicone mold or cake pan before air frying at 300F for 18-20 minutes until fudgy. Use a pan for cake and quickbread slices.

The air fryer's convection current gives fried ice cream a facelift. Roll ice cream balls in crispy cereal coating then place in freezer for 1-2 hours. Air fry coated balls at 300F for 5-7 minutes until outer layer crisps. Top with fruit sauce!

Traditional pineapple fritters turn out juicy tender on the inside with an airy crisp shell when air fried. Toss pineapple chunks in batter and air fry in a single layer for 8-10 minutes at 400F until golden.

Make churro apple fritters by slicing apples, tossing in cinnamon-sugar churro batter and air frying until crispy. For bananas foster fritters, coat banana slices in a sweet batter with rum extract then air fry.

Customize cake mixes by swapping oil for applesauce or yogurt before air frying according to box directions. The results are incredibly moist thanks to the circulating hot air.

Sheet cakes are perfect for the air fryer's compact space. Make confetti cake, marble cake or carrot cake in a small rimmed baking pan. Test for doneness with a toothpick.

The possibilities are endless for elevating typically "bad-for-you" guilty pleasures into healthier renditions with your air fryer's assistance. Satisfy cravings for sweets through creative cake, cookie and doughnut recipes cooked to crispy, fudgy perfection.

Low-Carb Cakes and Cookies

While the air fryer diet reduces sugar intake substantially, you can still occasionally enjoy slimmed-down sweet treats. The air fryer's convection heat bakes up incredible low-carb cake and cookie options with a fraction of the carbs. With clever substitutions, your favorite desserts can be transformed into guilt-free delights.

Starting with cakes, using almond or coconut flour rather than white flour eliminates most carbs right off the bat. While less absorbent, adding a bit more leavening agent helps these low-carb flours rise sufficiently. Cutting back on sugar and adding zucchini, pumpkin, or apple sauce keeps cakes moist. Icing or frosting is optional – fresh berries add sweetness with fiber.

An easy vanilla cake uses almond flour, baking powder, vanilla extract and eggs for lift. Coconut flour works for chocolate versions along with cocoa powder. Spices like cinnamon and nutmeg enhance natural sweetness as do sugar-free extracts. Serve frosted or unfrosted with whipped cream.

For pound cakes, substitute oil for butter and use heavy cream or nut milks to stay low carb. Try lemon poppyseed, marble or orange olive oil cakes. Bread flour helps provide lift once or twice weekly in moderation. Top slices with fresh sliced strawberries or peaches.

Cheesecakes are already lower carb and air fry beautifully for portion control. Beat cream cheese with eggs, lemon juice and vanilla then bake. An optional almond crust is tasty but not necessary. Garnish mini cheesecakes with fresh berries.

Mug cakes are a fast way to get your cake fix as a single serving. Find recipes using your favorite low-carb flours plus cocoa powder, berries, or other mix-ins blended right in the mug. The air fryer bakes these individual servings to fluffy perfection in under 10 minutes.

As for low-carb cookies, there are many formulations that come together quickly. Try recipes utilizing almond flour, coconut flour, flaxmeal or oat fiber as the flour base. Cut natural sweeteners like maple syrup and honey help keep carbs down.

Sneak extra nutrition into cookies by adding shredded zucchini or carrots, cocoa nibs, nut butter, and dark chocolate chips. Spices like ginger, cinnamon and nutmeg enhance chocolate and fruit flavors.

Some easy cookie options include chocolate chip, oatmeal raisin, coconut macaroons, peanut butter and lemon-blueberry thumbprints. Scoop dough onto a parchment lined air fryer basket. Bake at 325F for 7-9 minutes until set.

For grab-and-go breakfasts, make cookies more wholesome by incorporating protein powder, collagen or chia seeds into the dough. Or add nuts and dried fruit for an energy boost.

Cookie dough also transforms into quick breads like banana nut, zucchini or pumpkin loaves. Swap sugar for stevia or monk fruit-based sweeteners. The air fryer perfectly bakes individual servings by the slice.

While you'll still want to indulge in moderation, these slimmed-down takes on classic cakes and cookies help satisfy sweet cravings without sabotaging your diet goals. Be sure to promptly cool and store any leftover treats in the refrigerator or freezer to avoid overindulging.

Delicious Air Fryer Pies and Tarts

Pies and tarts are classic desserts, but traditional versions come packed with butter, oil and sugar. Luckily your air fryer allows you to recreate these sweet treats in a more nutritious way by reducing excess fat and calories.

Making mini fruit pies or petite tarts is an easy weeknight project or fun weekend baking activity. You control the ingredients so you can opt for less processed sugars and flours. The air fryer gives the same golden brown crust without all the added fat from frying.

Handheld Fruit Pies

Roll out refrigerated pie dough and cut into rounds with a biscuit cutter. Place sliced stone fruits like peaches, plums or apricots in the center. Fold dough over filling and crimp edges with a fork to seal. Cut slits on top and lightly brush with milk or egg wash. Air fry at 350F for 12-14 minutes until golden brown.

Sweet Potato Mini Tarts

Press small rounds of refrigerated sugar cookie dough into mini muffin tins and par-bake at 325F for 5 minutes. When cooled, fill with cubed roasted sweet potatoes, brown sugar, butter, cinnamon, and nutmeg. Top with more dough and air fry at 350F for 10-12 minutes until crust is set.

Pecan Pie Bars

Press refrigerated pie dough into a baking dish and par-bake for 5 minutes at 350F. In a bowl, mix brown sugar, vanilla, eggs, and chopped pecans. Pour filling over crust and return to air fryer for 15-18 minutes until set.

Rustic Galettes

Roll refrigerated pie dough into a circle. Pile sliced stone fruit in the center, leaving a 2-inch border. Fold border over fruit, pleating as needed. Brush with cream or milk and sprinkle sugar on top. Air fry at 350F for 20-25 minutes until browned and bubbly.

No-Bake Fruit Tarts

Press refrigerated sugar cookie dough into mini tart pans and air fry at 325F for 5-7 minutes until set. Fill cooled tart shells with instant vanilla or chocolate pudding. Top with fresh fruit like berries, kiwi, or mango.

Apple Hand Pies

Mix diced apples with brown sugar, cinnamon, lemon juice, and cornstarch. Place spoonfuls of filling onto dough rounds. Fold dough over apple mixture to form a half moon and crimp sealed edges. Air fry at 350F for 12-15 minutes.

Chocolate hazelnut Tart

Press chocolate cookie crumbs into a mini tart pan and air fry at 325F for 5 minutes. Fill with chocolate-hazelnut spread mixed with whipped cream. Top with chopped hazelnuts before serving.

With your air fryer you can reinvent classic desserts to align with your health goals. Using fresh fruit fillings and less fatty doughs allows you to indulge while still providing nutritional benefits. Get the whole family involved and let your air fryer work its magic for homemade pies and tarts in minutes.

Air Fryer Fruit Desserts

Thanks to its ability to caramelize and dehydrate, the air fryer brings out the natural sweetness in fruit to create healthy desserts. Take advantage of seasonal produce to make crisps, cobblers, fritters and more showcasing fruit's versatility.

For a quick dessert, air fry fruit with a topping like toasted oats, honey, coconut, granola or yogurt. Apples, pears, peaches, nectarines and apricots all shine when sliced and air fried until tender with a crispy coating.

Make apple and pear crisps by tossing sliced fruit with lemon, spices, sugar and flour. Top with an oat streusel mix then air fry at 375F until fruit bubbles and topping browns.

Cobblers take on new levels of flavorful caramelization when air fried. Prepare biscuit dough and press into the bottom of a pan. Top with sweetened fruit then air fry until dough is cooked through and fruit tender.

Poach fruit in flavors like wine, honey or fruit juice on the stovetop first before topping with batter and air frying for ultimate flavor infusion. Try wine-poached pears, honey-poached peaches or caramel apple fritters.

For more decadence, make skillet cakes and buckles by combining cake batter with fresh fruit before air frying to doneness in a skillet or pan. Enjoy classic flavor combos like pineapple upside down cake or blueberry buckle cake.

Hydrate dried fruits like apricots, cranberries, raisins or dates in hot liquid before mixing into batters and air frying for added moisture and sweetness. They make tasty additions to apple cakes, cranberry scones or fruit fritters.

Chunky fruit compotes are simple to prepare by air frying a combo of fruits like apples, berries, peaches, mangoes or pears with a splash of juice concentrate, honey or maple syrup. Serve warm or chilled over yogurt or ice cream.

Bake individual fruit galettes in ramekins or a mini pie pan crimped with dough and filled with a spiced fruit puree or fresh thinly sliced fruit. Brush crust with milk or egg wash before air frying until golden brown.

Make healthy fruit pizza for dessert by air frying prepared cookie dough into a crispy crust. Top with sweetened mascarpone or ricotta cheese and arrange fresh fruit slices artfully over top.

For belly-warming dessert, fill hollowed oranges, apples or pears with chopped dried fruits, nuts and spices. Drizzle with honey or maple syrup and air fry until fruit is tender.

The options are endless for experimenting with seasonal fruit in the air fryer. Enhance flavors through unique spice blends, herbs, extracts and sauces swirled into batter or poaching liquid. Let the air fryer coax out fruit's natural sugars for the perfect balance of sweet and tart.

CHAPTER 7

PLANNING YOUR MEALS FOR A BALANCED DIET

Essential Tips for Meal Planning

Meal planning is an essential habit for maintaining any healthy diet, especially the air fryer diet. Taking time to plan out nutritious meals and prep ingredients in advance saves time, money and sanity during busy weeks. This chapter will provide key tips for effortless weekly meal planning.

The first step is taking inventory of which healthy proteins, fresh produce, smart carbs and other staple ingredients you already have on hand. Check dates and use up anything that's close to expiring first. Make a list of needs for upcoming recipes to minimize food waste.

Next, browse air fryer cookbooks or online recipe sources and curate a variety of breakfasts, main dishes and sides you would enjoy making that week. Focus on dishes featuring the lean proteins, ample produce and whole grain sides emphasized in the air fryer diet.

Aim for a mix of quick weeknight meals as well as more complex dishes you can prepare in bigger batches on weekends. NEVER REPEAT main ingredients in the same week for maximum variety and nutrition. You can, however, repurpose leftovers into new meals later in the week.

When planning dinners, choose recipes that use overlapping main ingredients or components. For example, pick meals featuring ground turkey or chicken twice that week, allowing you to cook a double batch to use in both dishes. Or select sides that use the same veggie or grain base.

Overlap in seasonings and aromatics across meals also minimizes waste and preparation time. For instance, plan multiple dishes calling for garlic, onions, chili powder or other spices. Repurpose leftovers into snacks, salads or sides for a head start on future meals.

Make a detailed master grocery list to purchase all needed ingredients for the week in one single trip. Shopping with a planned list prevents impulse purchases that can derail your diet. Buy fresh produce at optimal ripeness unless meal prepping recipes in advance.

When it comes to actual cooking, the air fryer makes preparing multiple components of a meal fast and easy. You can air fry proteins, vegetables and side dishes simultaneously. For more elaborate meals, utilize the weekends to prep ingredients or sauces ahead of time.

Cleaning as you go also makes weekly meal prep less daunting. Hand wash used utensils and prep bowls quickly to prevent overwhelming messes. Plan out which nights will yield leftovers to reheat or repurpose so your weeknights are freed up as much as possible.

Meal planning tips:

- Browse new air fryer recipes weekly for inspiration

- Inventory ingredients on hand before grocery shopping

- Create a master grocery list to shop efficiently

- Plan a week's worth of varied, overlapping menus

- Prep bulk proteins, grains or cooked ingredients in advance

- Reuse leftovers creatively later in the week

- Prep produce as needed to maximize freshness

- Clean as you go to prevent messes

To save even more time, double batch meal components that freeze well. Cooked proteins, grains or chopped produce can be frozen for future recipes. Prepare a couple freezer meals fully assembled to reheat on busier nights.

Use your weekends wisely to cook 2-3 bigger batch meals you can portion out for quick lunches or dinners later on. For example, make a whole roasted chicken to use in tacos, sandwiches, soups and salads that week.

Take advantage of days off to make snacks or treats in advance too. This avoids needing to cook daily. Chop veggies for quick grab-and-go snacks. Or bake up a batch of air fryer granola bars, energy bites or chia pudding cups.

Following proper meal planning habits weekly is essential for maintaining the air fryer diet for the long haul. With an organized plan and prepped ingredients on hand, you set yourself up for diet success all week long!

Creating a Weekly Air Fryer Menu

Planning out a weekly menu is one of the best ways to set yourself up for air fryer cooking success. Taking time on the weekends to map out meals for the week ahead helps ensure you have healthy ingredients ready to go and alleviates the daily dinner dilemma.

Think through your schedule for the upcoming week - what days will be busier than others? When might you eat out or get takeout? How many dinners do you need to prepare at home?

With your week in mind, create an air fryer meal plan that includes variety and balance. Try to incorporate different proteins, plenty of vegetables, and both lighter and heartier dishes.

Focus first on utilizing ingredients you already have at home. Peruse your pantry and make a list. Seeing what staples you have on hand can spark recipe ideas and reduce food waste.

Then make your grocery list for any supplemental items needed for your menu. Shop for ingredients all at once over the weekend to minimize trips to the store throughout the week.

Here are some tips for building an air fryer meal plan:

- Vary cooking methods - include both from-scratch and shortcut options like using rotisserie chicken.

- Mix up global cuisines to add exciting new flavors.

- Find recipes that repurpose leftovers later in the week.

- Balance weekday convenience with more involved weekend meals.

- Add veggies to every dinner - roast, steam, air fry as sides.

- Keep weeknight dinners simple with salads, fajitas, sheet pan meals.

- Utilize your freezer - thaw proteins gradually during the week.

- Prep ingredients on weekends to allow for quick weeknight assembly.

- Make extra servings of entrees to use for weekday lunches.

Here is a sample weekly air fryer dinner menu:

- Monday: Apricot Glazed Pork Chops, Roasted Broccoli & Carrots

- Tuesday: Blackened Fish Tacos with Pineapple Salsa & Cilantro Lime Rice

- Wednesday: Crispy Chicken Thighs with Green Beans and Baked Potatoes

- Thursday: Zucchini Lasagna Rollups with Side Salad

- Friday: Steak Fajitas with Peppers and Onions, Guacamole & Chips

- Saturday: Teriyaki Salmon with Asparagus & Coconut Rice

- Sunday: Breaded Eggplant Parmigiana Sandwiches with Zucchini Fries

Planning ahead takes the guesswork out of dinner time and sets you up to stick with your air fryer diet all week long. Make meal prepping efficient by utilizing leftovers and stocking up on versatile ingredients. Follow your menu for stress-free healthy dinners your whole family will love.

Shopping Tips for Budget-Friendly Meals

One of the air fryer's perks is the ability to transform budget-friendly ingredients into delicious meals. With some savvy shopping strategies, you can keep costs low while enjoying a diverse array of air fried dishes. Follow these tips to get more value from every grocery run.

Stick to buying ingredients in their whole, unprocessed forms whenever possible. Whole foods like produce, grains, proteins and dairy generally cost less than pre-packaged and prepared items. You also control the quality and freshness.

Stock up on versatile base ingredients to use across many recipes, like eggs, onions, garlic, potatoes, carrots, beans, rice, herbs and spices. Build meals around what's already on hand to limit new specialty purchases per recipe.

Plan meals around in-season produce when flavors peak and costs drop. The air fryer excels at roasting vibrant veggies like summer's zucchini, squash and eggplant or fall's Brussels sprouts and sweet potatoes.

Purchase family packs or bulk values packs of meat and poultry, then portion and freeze extras in recipe-ready servings. The air fryer cooks smaller amounts of meat perfectly.

Canned, frozen and shelf-stable ingredients stretch dollars while providing convenience. Keep canned veggies, beans, tuna, tomatoes and fruit on hand along with frozen veggies, shrimp and lean ground meats.

Shop store brands, bulk bins and discount grocers for the best value on pantry staples like grains, oils, spices, condiments and baking ingredients. Avoid paying premium prices for national brands.

Scan weekly ads and load digital coupons before grocery trips. Combine sale prices with coupons on shelf-stable items to stock up at the lowest price.

Take advantage of weekly meat and produce sales, then build meals around those fresh ingredients. Marinate marked-down meat cuts in the air fryer for succulent dishes.

Don't overlook frozen foods when aiming for budget meals. The air fryer cooks many frozen foods exceptionally well, saving prep time. Try frozen fruits, vegetables, fish fillets and lean ground proteins.

Repurpose leftovers creatively into new air fried meals later in the week. Shred leftover chicken into wraps or toss extra veggies into egg scrambles or frittatas.

Grow your own herbs and vegetables when possible. Air fry dishes taste incredible accented with just-picked parsley, thyme, onions or peppers right from your garden.

Consider buying whole chickens or roasts and breaking them down into smaller cuts yourself. Uncooked chicken parts cost significantly less than packaged boneless cuts.

Substitute affordable nutritious starches like potatoes, sweet potatoes, beans, or lentils in place of pricier ingredients in recipes. The air fryer makes them irresistibly crispy.

With smart shopping habits and meal planning strategies, creating budget-friendly dishes with the air fryer is totally achievable. Let flavors, nutrition and savings motivate your grocery choices.

Portion Control and Meal Prep Ideas

Proper portion sizes and advance meal prep are key pillars for success on the air fryer diet. Controlling portions prevents overeating while prepping ingredients or full recipes in advance saves time and reduces temptation. This chapter explores slimming strategies for plate proportions and batch cooking.

When it comes to portions, use the "plate method" as a guide. Fill half your plate with non-starchy vegetables, a quarter with lean protein and a quarter with complex carbs like beans, lentils or whole grains. This ensures you get sufficient produce along with modest protein and smart carb portions.

Use measuring cups and food scales until you train your eyes and stomach to recognize proper amounts. Stick to fist-sized portions of proteins, a cupped handful of carbs, and at least 2 cups of vegetables or salad at meals. The air fryer's smaller capacity also prevents cooking large amounts.

When determining portions, be sure to account for any cooking fats or oils added. Even healthy fats like olive or avocado oil are calorie dense. Overdoing healthy fats can stall weight loss even if the rest of your meal is low carb.

For calorie dense foods like nuts, nut butters, cheese, avocado and oils, pay close attention to serving sizes. Pre-portion these foods into snack bags or containers for grab-and-go ease. This prevents mindlessly overeating.

Meal prepping proteins, grains and produce in advance allows for quick assembly of balanced meals throughout the week. Chop vegetables and pre-cook grains on weekends to use in meals and sides all week long.

Roast batches of chicken breasts, fish fillets, tofu or tempeh to use in bowls, salads, wraps or grain bowls. Cooked proteins keep well for 3-5 days refrigerated. Slice grilled meats for easy sandwiches or wraps.

Prep produce soon after purchase to prevent spoilage. Wash, dry, chop and store veggies in containers ready to pull for recipes or snacks. Precut fruits as well. Blanching or roasting vegetables in advance cuts down on cooking time.

Efficiently use leftover proteins, veggies and whole grains in new dishes later in the week. Transform roasted chicken into enchiladas, stir fries or noodle bowls. Roasted veggies blend into frittata or soup. Cooked grains make excellent salad topping. Repurpose wisely.

Take advantage of days off to prepare multiple meals at once. Braise chicken thighs or cook a roast along with veggies to use throughout the week. Make double batches of chili, soup or casseroles to freeze individual portions.

Prepping healthy snacks in advance also promotes portion control while saving time. Air fry batches of veggie chips, energy bites or coconut shrimp. Whip up chia puddings, overnight oats or boiled eggs for easy grab-and-go options.

Here are more meal prepping tips:

- Cook extra proteins to use in salads, grain bowls, wraps, etc.

- Roast sheets of vegetables to add to meals or snacks

- Make healthy dips and dressings to portion out

- Cook 2-3 larger batch meals on weekends

- Prepare multiple side dishes or bases like grains and beans

- Clean and chop produce when purchased for recipes

- Portion snacks like nuts, cheese and nut butters

- Assemble freezer-friendly meals to reheat later

Proper portioning takes practice, so use measuring tools until you learn to eyeball serving sizes. Prepping in advance normalizes healthier habits while saving money and time. With planning, you can control portions and prep like a pro!

Overcoming Common Meal Planning Challenges

Creating a weekly meal plan seems like an easy way to stay on track with healthy home cooking. But frustrations can arise that derail your best intentions and leave you reaching for takeout menus.

Don't let bumps in the road shake your resolve! With some simple strategies, you can troubleshoot common meal planning challenges. Stay committed to your air fryer diet by getting creative to solve issues as they pop up.

Not Knowing What to Make

Recipe inspiration evaporates by midweek, and you find yourself asking "What should I cook tonight?" Flip through air fryer cookbooks and pin recipes you want to try. Browse social media and food blogs for video tutorials on techniques. Maintain a running grocery list on your phone of meal ideas to spark creativity when you go blank.

No Time to Cook

Lengthy recipes get deprioritized on busy weeknights. Opt for dishes with short prep times that utilize your air fryer's efficiency. Marinate proteins the night before. Do some chopping on weekends and store prepped ingredients. Rely on pantry staples like eggs, canned beans, frozen veggies.

Picky Eaters in Your Family

It's frustrating when the dinners you painstakingly plan get rejected. Involve family members in meal decisions and prep. Let kids customize their plates from interchangeable components. Offer two choices for finicky eaters. And serve new foods alongside familiar dishes to ease into variety.

Recipe Boredom Sets In

Tired of rotating the same meals? Infuse excitement by exploring new cuisines. Find air fryer cookbooks focused on regional or international fare. Let unique ingredients and global flavors renew inspiration.

You Fall Off Track

A crazy week derails even the best meal plan. Get back on track with a fridge clean-out meal using leftovers. Make a large batch of chili or soup to eat for several days. Keep frozen pizzas or nuggets on hand for emergencies. Be gentle with yourself when life happens - just get back to it when you can.

Grocery Shopping Dilemmas

Despite vigilance, you still forget key ingredients or get home to discover something spoiled. Make a master grocery list on your phone that you tweak each week. Keep staples like eggs, frozen veggies, rice stocked up. Shop midweek to replenish perishables.

By troubleshooting frustrations and building in contingencies, you can stick to your healthy meal plan despite hurdles. Be patient and persistent - with time, planning nutritious air fryer meals will get easier. Don't let challenges derail your progress. With some creativity, you've got this!

Tracking Your Progress

Embarking on the air fryer diet requires adjusting your mindset, habits and relationship with food. To ensure lasting success, make self-monitoring and progress tracking integral parts of your journey. Measure both objective data and subjective experiences to maximize results.

Begin by establishing clear baseline metrics before starting the diet. Record your current weight, body measurements, blood pressure, blood sugar or cholesterol levels. Calculate your daily caloric intake and nutritional breakdown. This provides concrete data to compare against as you advance.

Weigh yourself weekly under consistent conditions, like mornings before eating or drinking. Note your weight along with body measurements if desired. Avoid daily weigh-ins, as normal fluctuations may discourage you. Focus on the overall downward trend.

Keep a food log to increase self-awareness of what, when and how much you eat each day. Jot down meals, snacks, ingredients, cooking methods, portion sizes and hunger cues. Review patterns weekly. Digital food trackers can also help.

Calculate nutritional intake weekly to ensure you're meeting health needs while running a calorie deficit. Get sufficient protein, fiber, vitamins and minerals. Adjust if certain nutrients fall consistently low.

Record exercise habits like minutes spent doing cardio, strength training or activity types. Gradually increase duration and intensity. Pair food logs with exercise logs to understand your energy expenditure.

Beyond objective metrics, track subjective experiences in a journal. Note energy levels, sleep quality, mood, sugar cravings, joint pain or other symptoms. Identify lifestyle factors that influence your wellbeing.

Monitor how the diet affects your digestion, immunity and mental clarity over time. Check that you're consuming enough calories and nutrients to support healthy bodily functions.

Pay attention to cues of hunger and fullness so you can refine portion sizes accordingly. Note circumstances, times of day and triggers leading to cravings so you can start identifying patterns.

Click progress pictures weekly in similar clothing and poses. The visual changes will often be more dramatic than the numbers on the scale. Pictures keep you motivated.

Schedule regular check-ins with your doctor or dietitian to assess lab work and discuss successes or areas for improvement. Revise your plan based on expert insights.

Be consistent in your tracking efforts, but flexible. Life happens - don't abandon all progress if you have an indulgent vacation or a hectic workweek throws you off course. Just get back on track.

Consistency breeds habits. As weighing, measuring, logging and checking in becomes routine, you'll gain clarity on how to nourish your body optimally. Let data guide you toward your health and weight loss goals.

CONCLUSION

Embracing an air fryer diet opens up a world of possibilities for making over your favorite comfort foods in a healthier way. By utilizing this innovative appliance, you can cut back on excess fat, calories, and processed ingredients while still enjoying all the flavors and textures you crave.

With an air fryer, gone are the days of deep frying everything in batches of oil. This more nutritious cooking method significantly reduces added fats and eliminates exposure to potentially dangerous acrylamides that form in overheated oils. Who wouldn't want to ditch the greasy mess for faster, cleaner cooking?

The benefits extend far beyond cutting calories though. Using your air fryer encourages you to cook more dishes from wholesome scratch ingredients. With so many tempting recipes at your fingertips, you can give nearly any takeout or restaurant favorite a homemade makeover. Quick weeknight dinners have never been easier.

Cooking at home more frequently also saves money compared to buying pre-packaged and processed convenience items. And when you prepare dishes yourself, you control exactly what goes into your food. Skipping mystery ingredients allows you to focus on nutritional quality.

Following an air fryer diet provides health advantages for the whole family as well. Exciting new flavors will tempt even picky eaters to expand their palates. Kids can get involved helping with meal prep. And enjoying home cooked dinners together offers a chance to unwind and connect at the end of busy days.

Of course, changing eating habits requires an adjustment period. Be patient with yourself as you learn new dishes and techniques. Start by substituting air fried options for fried takeout favorites. Over time, you will discover just how versatile this appliance can be.

Don't let minor setbacks derail your progress. Each small change brings you one step closer to your goals. Remember to celebrate little victories along the way.

With some creativity and commitment, an air fryer diet can transform your health and relationship with food for the better. The initial investment will pay dividends for years to come in the form of more energy, steady weight loss, and an overall healthier lifestyle.

If you seek convenience without compromising nutrition, let this handy appliance revitalize your cooking. Equipped with an arsenal of tempting recipes, you can finally stop missing out on fried deliciousness. Embrace this better-for-you cooking method and never look back!

BONUS 1

12 VIDEO TUTORIAL RECIPES

Scan the QR code

BONUS 2

6 AMAZING STEP-BY-STEP RECIPES

Scan the QR code

Darren Carr

BONUS 3

45 FULL RECIPES TUTORIALS

Scan the QR code

BONUS 4

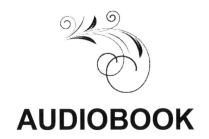

AUDIOBOOK

Scan the QR code and download the MP3 files to listen to the audiobook

EXCLUSIVE BONUS

3 EBOOK

Scan the QR code or click the link and access the bonuses

http://subscribepage.io/01tYl3

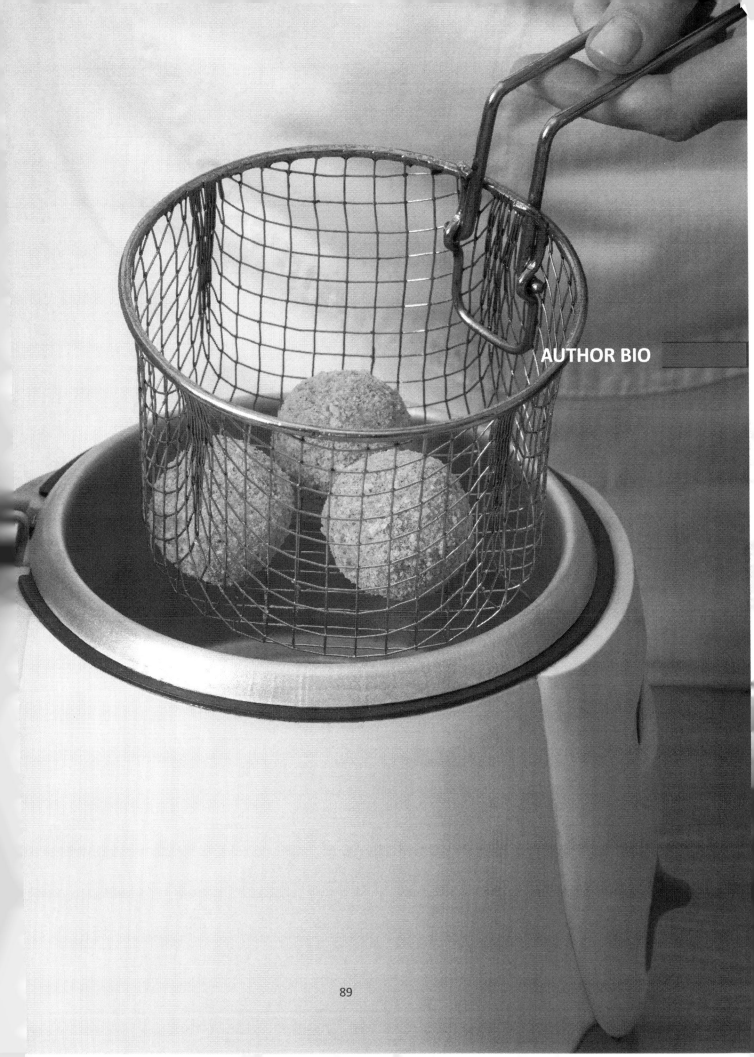

Darren Carr

Darren Carr is a passionate food and culinary expert whose life has been a journey of culinary exploration and discovery of gastronomic delights. Growing up in a family environment where cooking was at the center of daily life, Carr cultivated a deep passion for the world of flavors and food preparations from a young age.

After completing his culinary studies and working in renowned restaurants, Darren embarked on culinary trips to different parts of the world, studying the culinary traditions of different cultures. He learned from celebrity chefs and culinary masters, honing his skills in preparing sophisticated and palate-pleasing dishes.

Darren Carr is also a devoted father and husband. His family shares his love of food and they often spend time together cooking and experimenting with new recipes.

Printed in Great Britain
by Amazon